BODYWEIGHT EXERCISES FOR WOMEN

Simple Exercises to Help you Lose Weight and Sculpt your Body

Andy Charalambous

Contributors To This Book

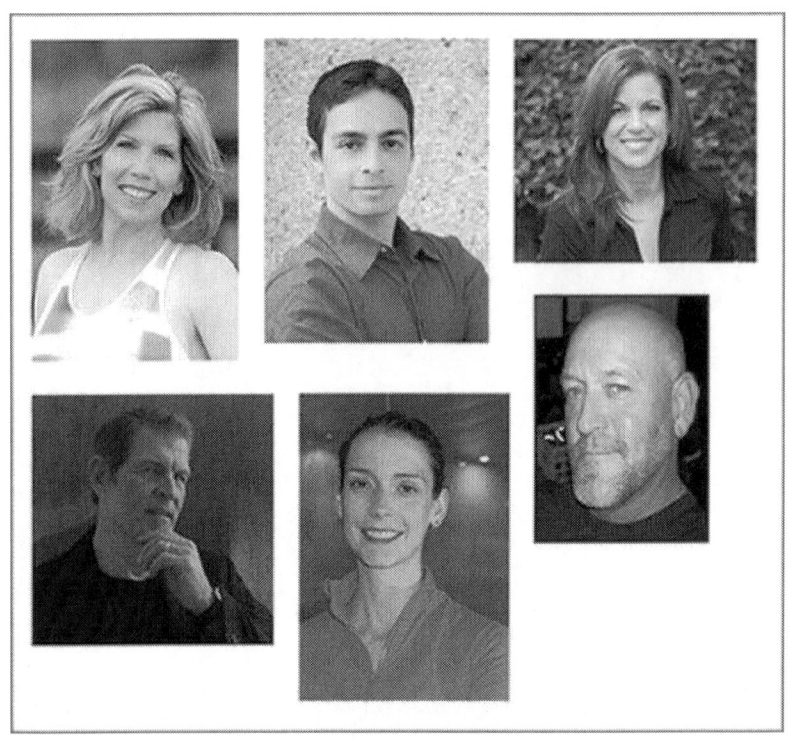

FIT EXPERT SERIES

FREE GIFTS!

THIS BOOK IS PACKED WITH FREEBIES!

Igor Klibanov is giving away 2 gifts! **$319** Worth of Pure Body-Changing, Performance-Enhancing Information and also his "Fat Loss for the Mature, Confident Woman" book. READ HIS CHAPTER FOR DETAILS.

Nicole LaBonde is giving you **FREE ACCESS** to her Cabarret video, "The Thigh Toning Booty Blasting Leg Series".
READ HER CHAPTER FOR DETAILS.

Steve Payne is giving away **FREE** reports on virtually every aspect of fitness success.
READ HIS CHAPTER FOR DETAILS.

DON'T MISS OUT!

Copyright Information

Bodyweight Exercises For Women
By
Andy Charalambous
Copyright 2013 Andy Charalambous

You agree to hold the Author of this Book, the Author's owners, agents, co-authors, contributors, affiliates and employees harmless from any and all liability for all claims for damages due to injuries, including attorney fees and costs incurred by you or caused to third parties by you, arising out of the products, services and activities discussed in this Book.

Fact and information are believed to be accurate at the time they were placed in this Book. All data provided in this Book is to be used for information purposes only. Information provided is not all-inclusive and is limited to information that is made available and such information should not be relied upon as all-inclusive or accurate.

Recommended Related Books

More Books you may like by Andy Charalambous

Just type 'Andy Charalambous' in the Amazon search bar to see all of his latest books:

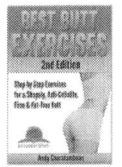 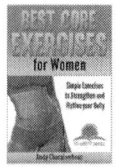 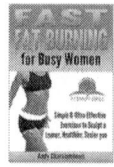 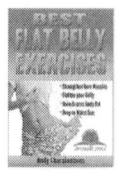 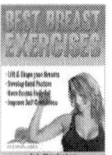

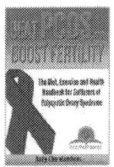 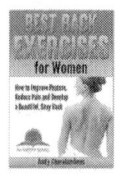 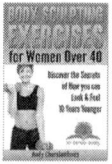 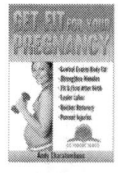 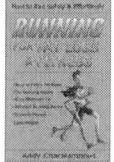

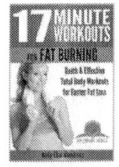 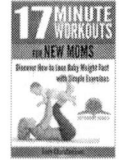 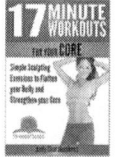 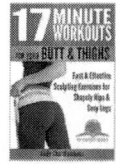 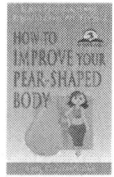

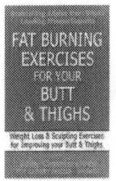 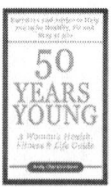 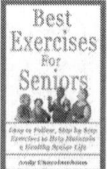 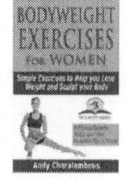 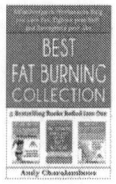

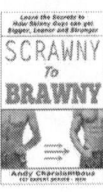 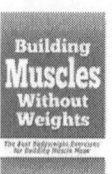 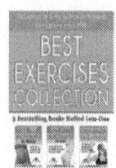 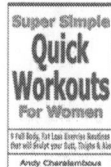

Introduction

Wouldn't it be great if we could be able to shape our bodies without having to set foot in a gym? Wouldn't it be great if we could just workout at home without having to use any kind of exercise equipment?

Well, this is very possible when incorporating bodyweight exercises into your routine.

In this book you have the opportunity to get the best advice from six professional fitness trainers. Each trainer has gone into detail explaining what they think you should be doing to achieve specific goals.

There are a number of exercise routines to follow, each designed to achieve a difinitive goal and help sculpt your body.

How many of you ladies hop from one exercise machine to the next when you are in the gym? I would bet quite a few of you are doing this. Ok, at least you are staying in motion which is a good thing but the truth is most of these machines tend to only isolate one muscle group. This would mean that you burn fewer calories and work less muscle as opposed to doing an exercise that works a number of muscle groups.

Ok, so what are bodyweight exercises? Basically these are a combination of strength training exercises and routines that do not require you to join a gym or use any kind of free weights.

These are specific exercises that have the practitioner use their own bodyweight to provide the resistance for the movements.

The popularity of this kind of training is growing for men and women and so there are so many movements available to use. Some of the more favoured moves are exercises such as the push-up, the pull-up and various kinds of core work supporting the abdominal area.

With this type of training you can workout pretty much anywhere and anytime at no extra expense. You don't need any additional food supplements or exotic "trending" exercise equipment. All you will need is the desire and motivation to improve yourself.

Having said that, for certain exercises weights can be incorporated to increase the difficulty of the workout. Also some exercises do require some sort of apparatus to lean on or hang from but these are not necessarily all located at the gym. You can improvise by using your surroundings.

For example, you could use a park bench to do a number of exercises including step-ups and triceps dips. You could use the top bar of a swing in a playground to do pull-ups. Anything is possible; just use your imagination.

Bodyweight exercises tend to require more flexibility and balance compared to using machines in the gym. This means these are perfect for women seeing as they tend to be more flexible than men.

You can progress or regress to meet your own personal needs. This strategy allows all ages and all levels of fitness to participate.
So whatever your fitness level, whatever your age, bodyweight exercises can work well for you. Just give them a try and you will not only see fast improvements but you will also have fun doing them.

Table of Contents

CHAPTER 1

Steve Payne

31 Days to a Better Butt, a Tighter Tummy and Awesome Arms

I'm a fitness professional living and working in San Antonio, Texas. I've been in the business a long time. And when I say a long time, I mean since the earth's crust was cooling...

I've worked with hundreds of women and I can state emphatically that each and every one of them wanted three simple things:

1. A better looking butt

2. A flatter stomach

3. Great looking arms

I'm quite certain you feel the same way as well.

Here's the conundrum...you don't like the thought of lifting weights, much less actually doing it, because you're afraid of getting bulky.

Am I right?

I'm going to put those fears to rest right here and now, once and for all.

Ready?

If your goal is a lean, sexy and trim overall appearance, at some point you need to perform heavier strength and resistance exercises during your training to get maximal results.

Unfortunately, most of the pictures of female bodybuilders have scared away every woman in the world from doing this, to their own detriment.

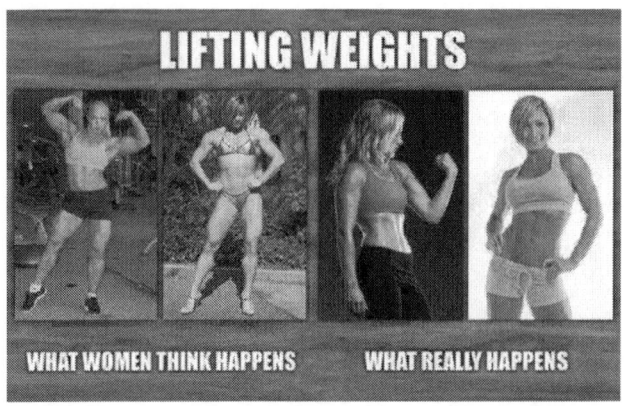

You will get superior results by performing HEAVIER resistance training, and I do not mean a few soup can sized dumbbell exercises at the end of your cardio routine. How do I know this...I mean, besides the fact that I've worked with hundreds of women for over 30 years?

Let me reiterate: Performing resistance based strength training exercises will make you leaner, sexier, hotter, more toned, feel better, look better and have more energy!

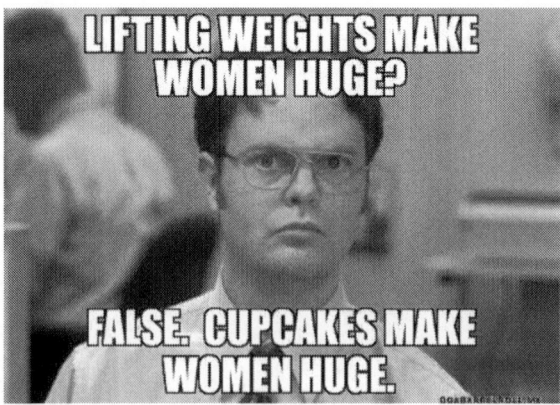

Now, just in case you don't believe me, here are 3 reasons lifting heavier weights **WILL NOT** make you bulky:

1. Some female bodybuilders on the cover of those magazines that you see in line at the grocery store take steroids. You aren't doing that.

2. Men naturally have 7-8x the concentration of testosterone that women do. How many men struggle to gain muscle? Probably the majority of the men you know. So, if they are struggling and have this supposed *significant* advantage, believe me when I say that you are not going to turn into she-hulk over night.

3. When you are building muscle, it is a slow process and it takes time. The body doesn't just pile on more tissue as soon as you touch a weight.

Are you convinced yet?

Just in case, here's another chilling fact for you: If you don't lift weights or perform resistance and strength exercises to gain muscle, every year after you turn 30, your body loses an average of 1lb of muscle which decreases the amount of calories you burn and leads to fat gain.

That's why so many women slowly gain weight as they get older. Just think…*GOODBYE SPANKS!*

And if gaining fat doesn't scare the bejeepers out of you then consider this: without performing strength and resistance training exercises that are challenging, your body slowly loses bone mass as well, and we all know this can lead to osteoporosis and osteopenia, the precursor to osteoporosis.

Here are 3 reasons why muscle will help you avoid that:

1. Muscle helps you burn more fat while at rest, which means you can eat more and not gain weight. (Hello carbs!) It's also a great thing for long term body composition maintenance.

3

2. Muscle just makes everything look better. Want that round butt? It all starts with well built glutes and hamstrings. Defined shoulders? You need to develop your deltoids. Muscle fills in all the areas that are supposed to be there and helps you burn off the things that aren't supposed to be there.

3. Being stronger helps you to prevent osteoporosis and osteopenia.

And since muscle is not limited to just the portions of the body you can see, having quality muscle means better digestion through more efficient peristalsis, a healthy and strong heart means better heart rate, breathing becomes more easily accomplished because of stronger diaphragmatic muscles and core strength and posture is enhanced.

So what does this mean to you? Building muscle should be your primary goal for achieving the body you want.

Here's the bottom line: If you will work to acquire more muscle, you will get more lean and sculpted, prevent bone and muscle decay as you age. This is the best ANTI-AGING combo around.

You can perform a great deal of strength and resistance type movements with just your own body weight. However, in order to get the benefits, you must manipulate your training somewhat in order to achieve success.

How do we do this? We have several choices:

- Increase exercise volume (either by number of sets or repetitions)
- Increase exercise load (Adding some weight to our body like a weighted vest or backpack)
- Increase exercise time under tension (how long an exercise lasts per set)

4

- Increase exercise intensity (how vigorously you train)

- Increase or decrease the range of motion of an exercise

- Speed up or slow down the pace of an exercise

- Minimize the amount of rest between sets of exercise

- Increase duration of exercise time (my least favorite method)

- Pair and or "stack" exercises together (my personal favorite)

At the end of this chapter I will provide you with a complete 31 day exercise and training program that will get you a better butt, a tighter tummy and awesome arms, and you're going to earn them.

Why?

Because we live in the body we earn.

Are you ready?

A Better Butt

Before we get started on training, I would be remiss if I did not mention this one fact of looking great.

Are you ready for it?

Here it is: ***you cannot out train crappy eating habits.***

If you're looking to turn heads *in a good way* at the beach, you've got to be eating a high quality, nutrient dense, supportive nutrition diet. Anything less will give you lackluster results and you and I both know you deserve much better than that.

If you're not sure what you need to do, do a little research. Keep it simple and don't fall for all of the diet and nutrition hype and superfluous garbage. You do not need a bunch of supplements, pills or powders. The simplest eating plan I know comes straight from the hand of God. Here it is: If you can't pick it from a plant, tree or shrub, or if it doesn't run, fly or swim...don't eat it.

And don't drink your calories.

Should you perchance stumble across a tortilla tree or 7-Up river please call me. We'll eat and drink our fill. Until then, eat the real stuff.

Enough said.

I remember it like it was yesterday, although it was almost 15 years ago. I had a female client performing sets of lunges and she stated, "You sure seem to enjoy having me do lunges. Why is that?"

"Because in the 15 or so years I've been working with women, I've never once heard one of them proclaim, 'We don't need to work on my butt. It looks good enough as it is.'"

She didn't say another word. She just turned and started another set of lunges.

For this 31 day program, you'll be training 6 days per week, performing a select group of exercises in rapid succession, with a pretty high volume and a minimal of rest. It is a progressive program, which means each days training session will build from the last. You'll do a little more each day until it's over.

There's a lot of variety, and you shouldn't get bored or stagnate, so let's take a look at the exercises and how to best perform them. We'll go through these pretty quickly.

The Squat

I love the squat.

Simple, basic and effective...if done properly.

Envision the bottom of your foot. See the ball of the big toe, the ball of the little toe and the ball of the heel. Now picture these three points of contact as a tripod on the ground.

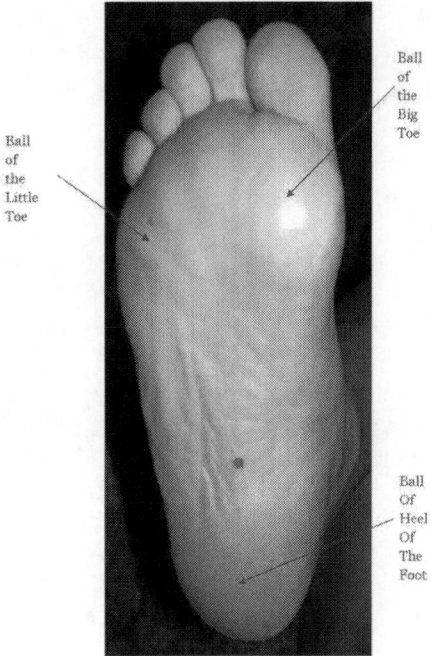

Ball of the Big Toe

Ball of the Little Toe

Ball Of Heel Of The Foot

Tripod Foot Description

When you do your squat, aside from making sure your range of motion is sound, this is all I want you to focus on; **keeping those three points of contact securely intact with the floor.**

Why?

Everything starts from the ground up on the squat. You cannot perform a squat poorly if and when those three points of contact are always on the floor.

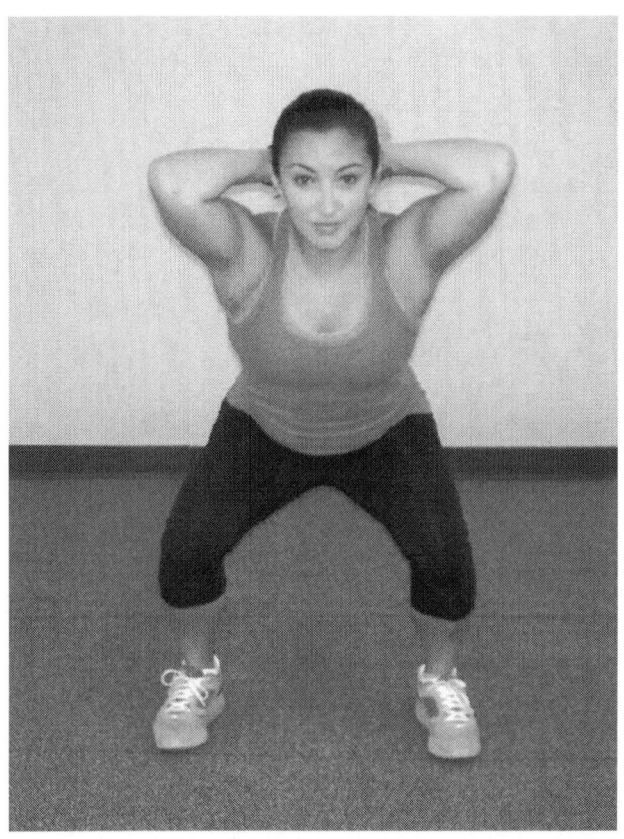

Squat Finish With Tripod Foot Position

If your knees cave inwardly, it could be because the ball of the little toe has come away slightly from the floor. Focus on the tripod and you may correct it.

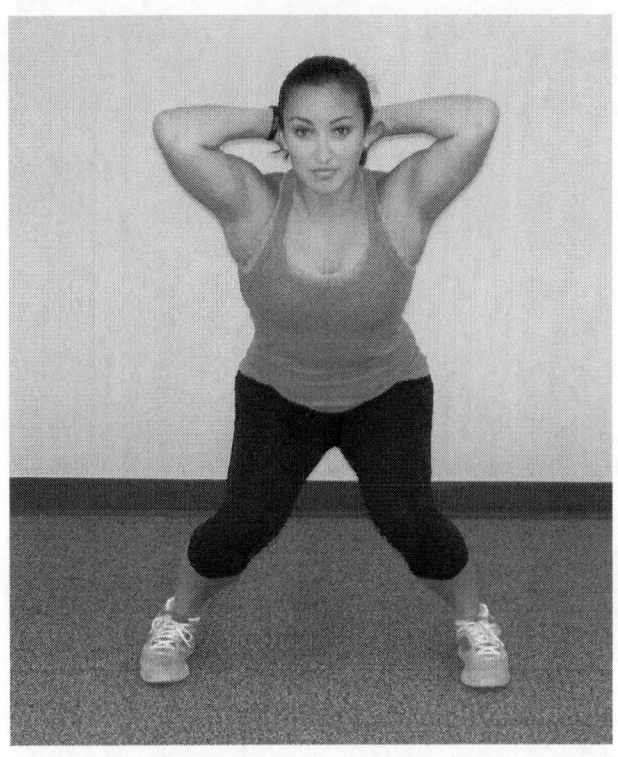

<u>Poor Squat Finish With Valgus Knee Position (Inward Caving)</u>

If your knees travel forward excessively, it is because the heel has risen from the floor.

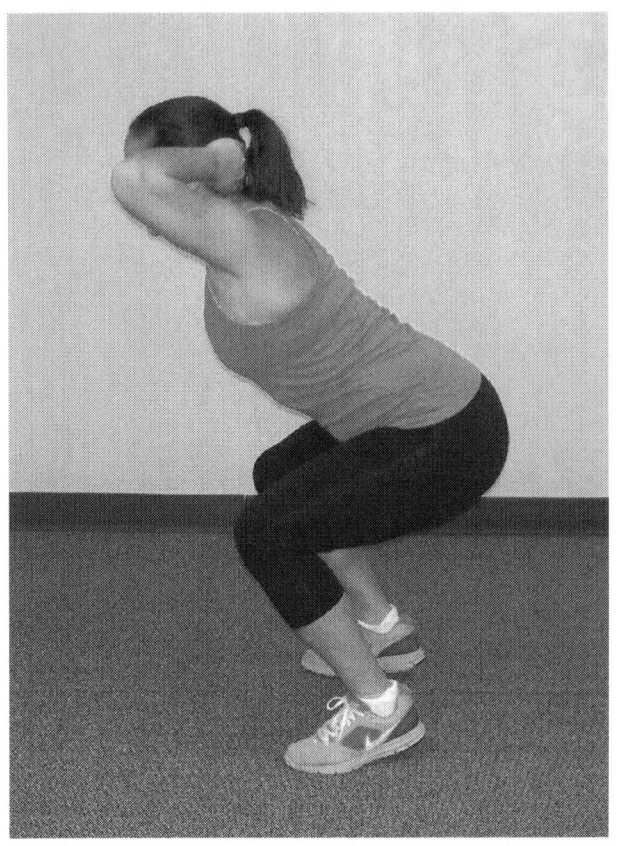

Poor Squat Finish With Heels Raised

Keep that tripod sound and everything else takes care of itself.

When you squat, try to drop your butt as near the floor as you can. If you experience pain in the knee, hip or back, stop just shy of the painful area. As I tell my clients, go to the point of pain, not through it. Also, go see someone and get that fixed. It isn't supposed to hurt.

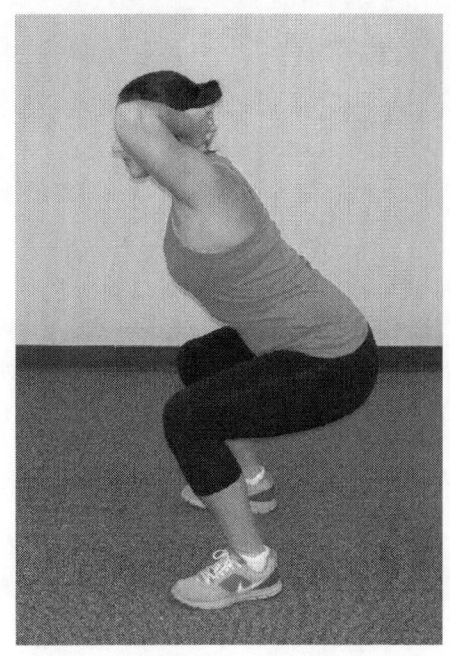

Prisoner Squat Finish Position with Hands Behind the Head

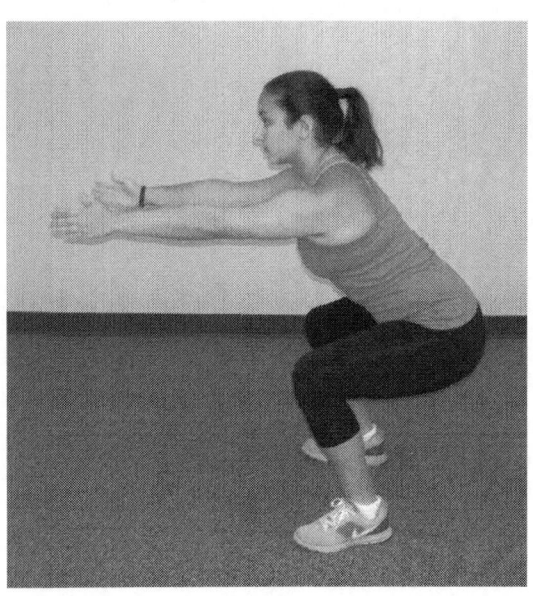

Keep your ribcage up and your chin parallel with the floor as you move. If you can place your hands behind your head and maintain an upright posture while squatting, do that. Otherwise hold your hands out in front of you for balance and stability.

The Shoulders Elevated Hip Lift (SEHL)

These can be performed from a bench, a sofa, the end of the bed or anywhere you can comfortably lay your shoulders and head.

Lie back on a secure surface so that the edge of your shoulders and head are comfortably resting on it. Place your feet in front of you so that when your hips are raised, your knees are bent at 90 degrees and your weight is on your heels.

Now, inhale gently and lower the hips until they are just off the floor, then, while driving through the heels, exhale and lift the hips until you have a straight line from your knees to your shoulders. Be sure to squeeze the glutes tight, but do not over extend or hyperextend the back.

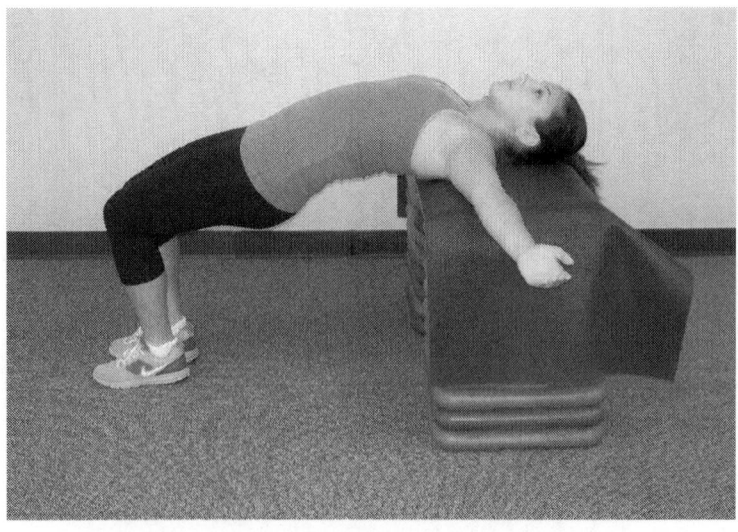

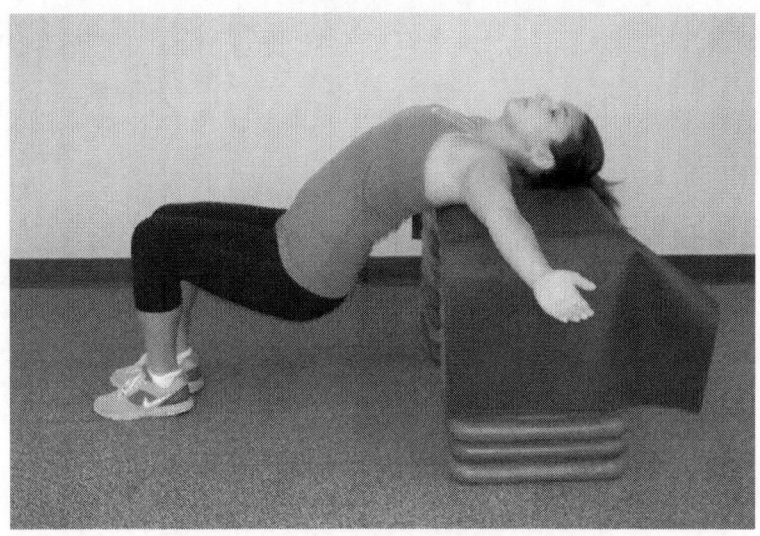

SEHL Start

The Reverse Lunge

The Reverse Lunge is a great butt development tool, but a few key points must be in order to be performed safely and effectively.

1. Maintain that tripod foot position on the forward leg at all times.
2. Step back under control to begin the reverse lunge exercise.
3. Drop the hips downward rather than let them float backwards during the exercise.
4. Keep the knee and the ankle of the forward leg in vertical alignment.
5. Keep the position of the rear foot vertical (heel pointed at the ceiling) with the knee slightly bent and just off the floor.
6. Keep the ribcage up and the chin parallel with the floor as much as possible during the movement.
7. Step forward under control and squeeze the glutes at the top of the movement.

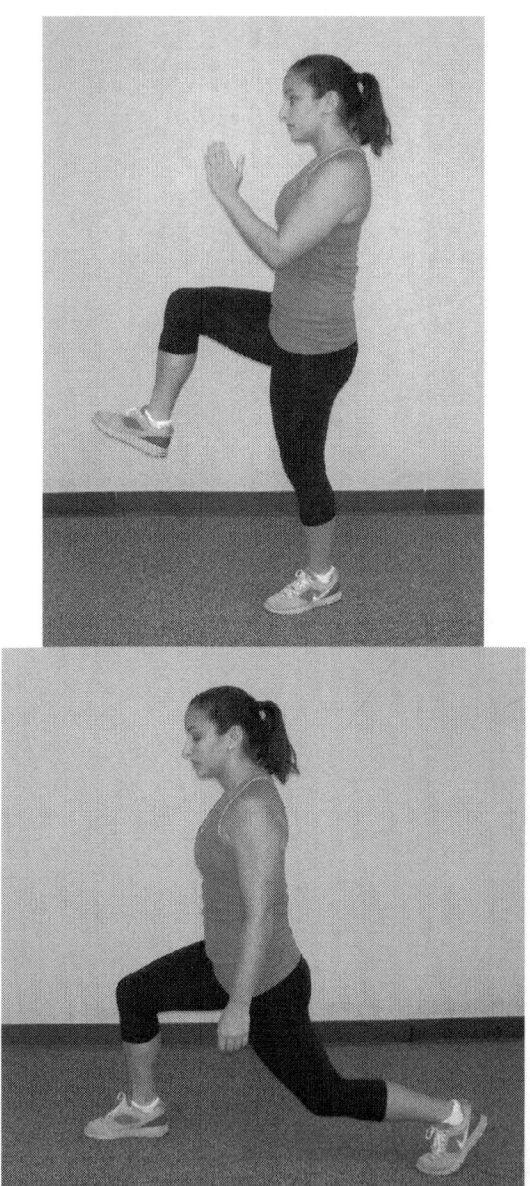

Reverse Lunge Position Start (left) and Finish (right)

Single Leg Shoulders Elevated Hip Lift (SLSEHL)

14

Perform this movement exactly like the Shoulders Elevated Hip Lift except on one leg.

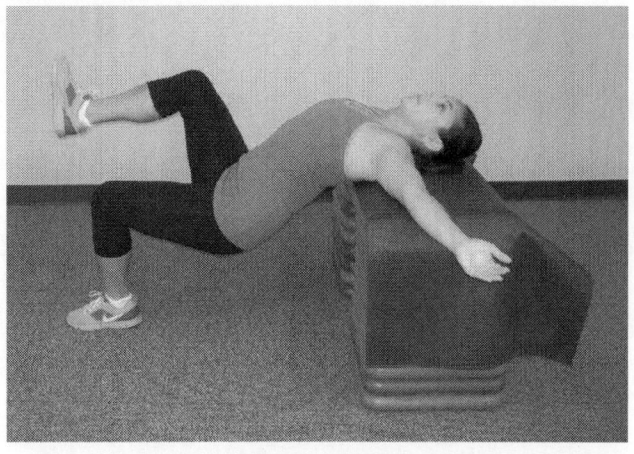

SLSEHL Start

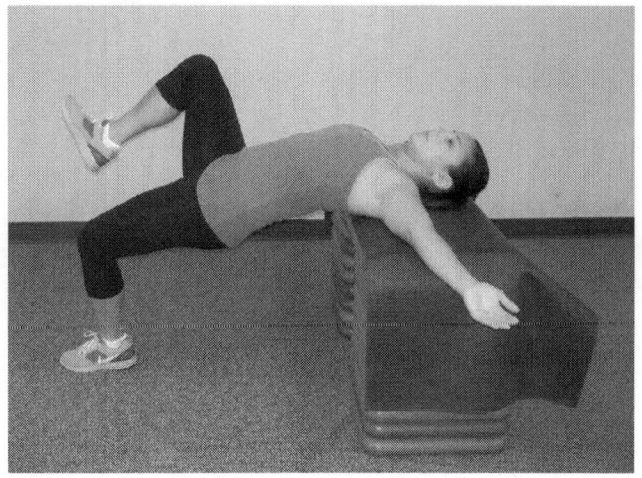

SLSEHL Finish

Draw the leg that is not doing the work into the chest as much as possible while performing the exercise. To increase the demand and intensity of the exercise, point it at the ceiling while doing it. To increase it even further, hold the leg out parallel to the floor while moving. Keep the hips parallel to the floor during the exercise.

15

Rear Foot Elevated Split Squats (RFESS)

These are frequently called Bulgarian Squats, but whatever you call them...they WORK!

You'll need a bench, stool or some surface upon which to place a foot while doing these exercises. The bench should be about the same height as your kneecap.

Standing in front of the bench approximately 2 feet (depending upon your reach, of course) extend one leg back until it is atop the bench.

Keep the front foot squarely on the floor in the tripod position, exhale and then under control, lower the hips to the floor. Make sure the ribcage is up and your chin is parallel with the floor.

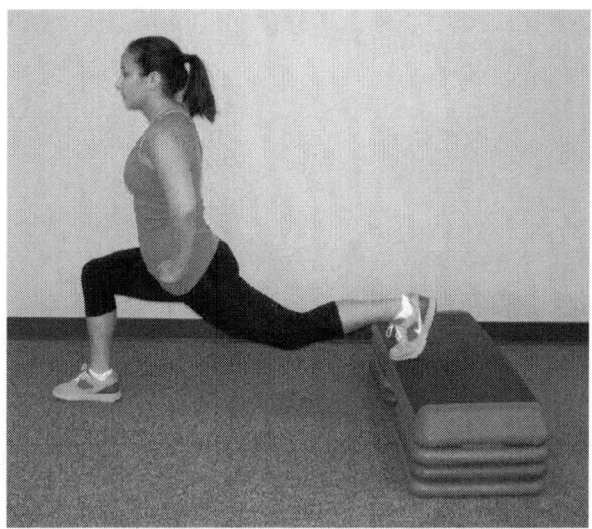

RFESS Start

You will feel a slight stress, stretch or pressure on the thigh of the rear leg, particularly if you're tight in that area. Move with as much range of motion as you are capable while maintaining good form.

Try to get the knee of the rear leg as close to the floor as possible, then exhale and drive the hips back to the start position, squeezing the glutes at the top.

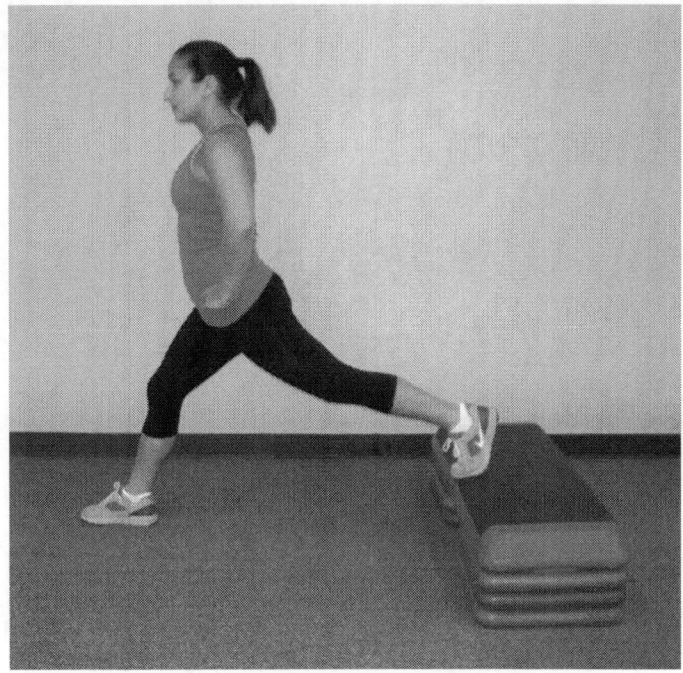

RFESS Finish

Hips Elevated Walk Outs (HEWO)

Lie on the floor and draw your feet in close to your butt. Place your weight on your heels and raise your hips.

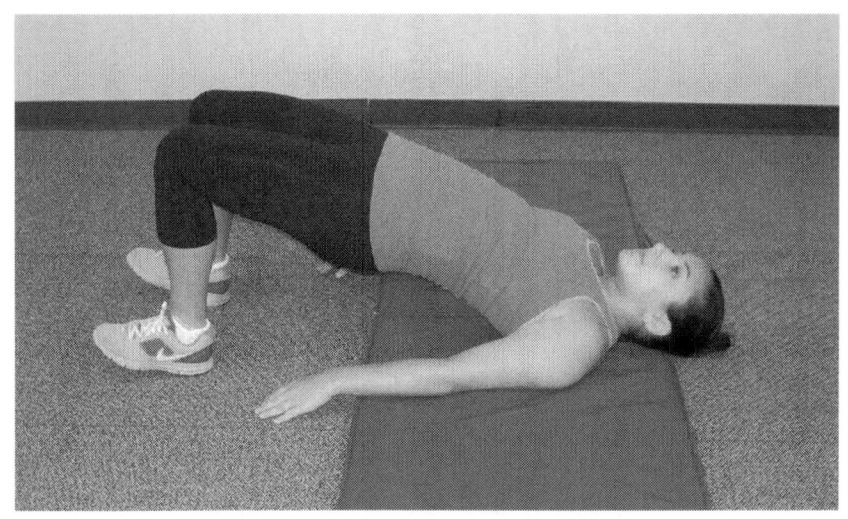

HEWO Beginning Position

Keeping the hips off the floor and walking on the heels, take small steps forward as far as you can without dropping the hips.

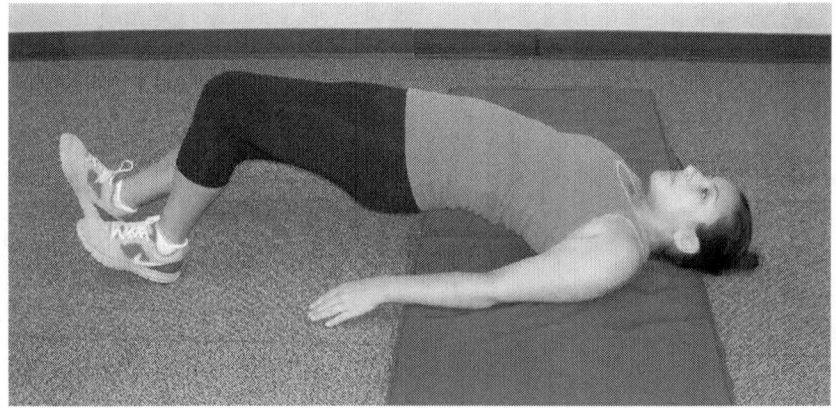

HEWO Ending Position

Walk the heels back to the start position under control.

Single Leg RDL (SLRDL)

We call these the "drinking bird" in my training sessions. If you're over the age of 45, you might remember them. If not, here's what they look like:

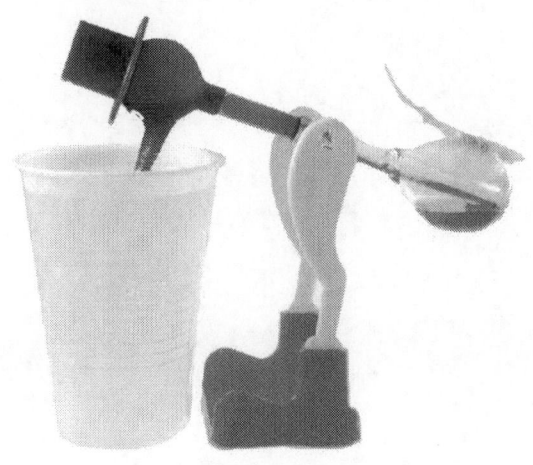

Such a happy little bird…

Please note where the pivot point is on this happy little bird.

Right in the hip. That's how you're going to move as well.

Place one foot in the tripod position on the floor and slightly bend the knee. For a thought, just think "soft knee" as you perform the movement.

Now squeeze the glute of the other leg and extend it slightly behind you.

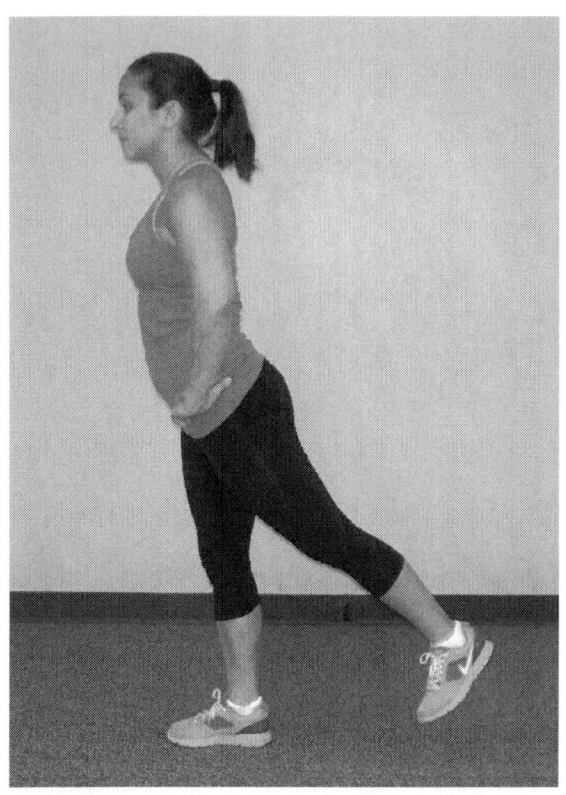

SLRDL Start Position With Glute Squeeze

Focus your gaze on a spot on the floor about 3 feet in front of you then, keeping the tripod squarely on the floor, act like a drinking bird and move your upper body and leg under control as a unit, bending forward at the hips. If you have trouble with your balance, place a small bench or stool in front of you to gently (but not rely on) lay a hand on for stability.

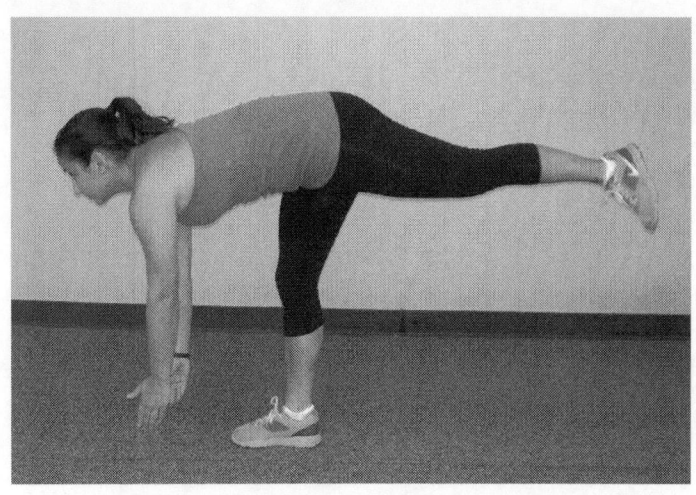

SLRDL End Position With Arms Down

Exhale and return to the start position. Remember to always squeeze the glute of the leg that is moving.

To make this exercise more challenging, extend the arms forward and pretend to reach for something across the room in front of you as you move.

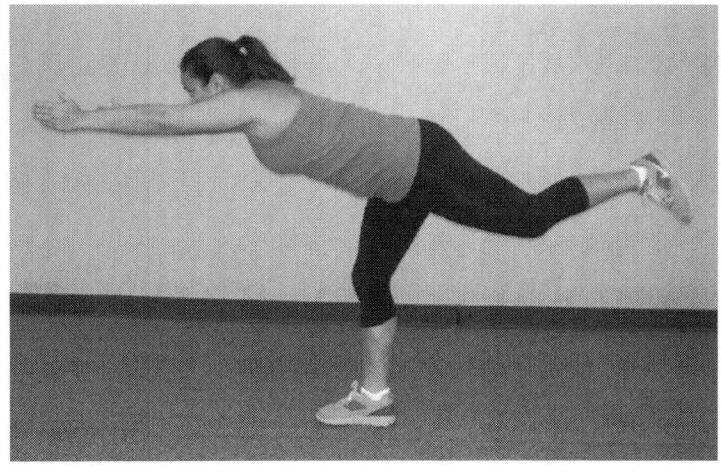

SLRDL With Arms Extended

Lying Band Resisted Hip Drives (LBRHD)

You'll need a resistance band of some sort, whether it's a piece of Theraband, a small training band or a full size 40 inch one. It doesn't need to be of great resistance, just enough to elicit some resistance to your movement.

Place a band across both legs, either directly above or below the kneecap. Either is fine; just find which position you prefer. Lie on your back on the floor with your feet far enough apart to place a minimum of resistance from the band against your legs. Draw both feet in close to your butt and drive through your heels until your hips come off the floor.

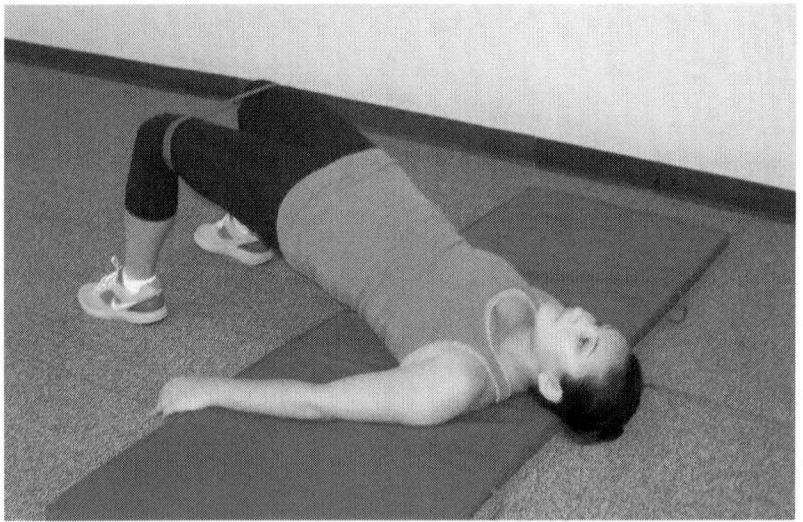

LBRHD Start

Keeping the hips elevated and weight on the heels, drive the knees outward under control a few inches, then return to the start position, but do not let the hips drop until the full set of the exercise is completed.

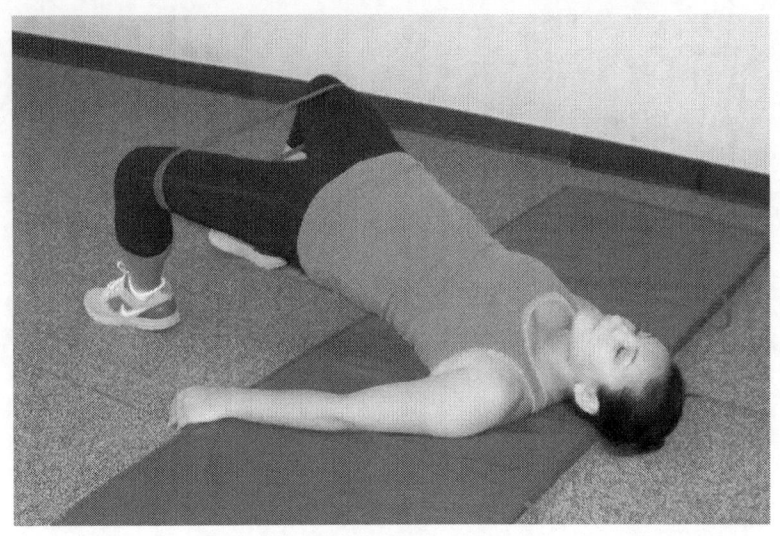

LBRHD Finish

"Pain In The Butt" Planks (PITBP)

Get into the front plank position, with the elbows positioned directly under the shoulders and your body makes a straight line from ankles to ears. Do not let the center of the back between the shoulder blades dip or the forehead drop as you do this.

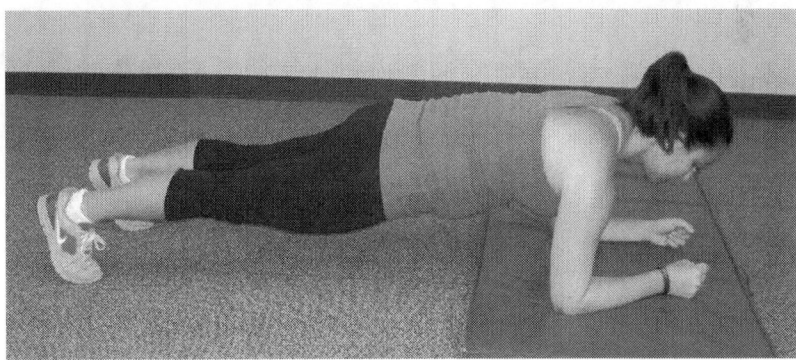

PITBP Good Start – Elbows Positioned Directly Under Shoulders, Head to Ankle Alignment and Scapula Flat

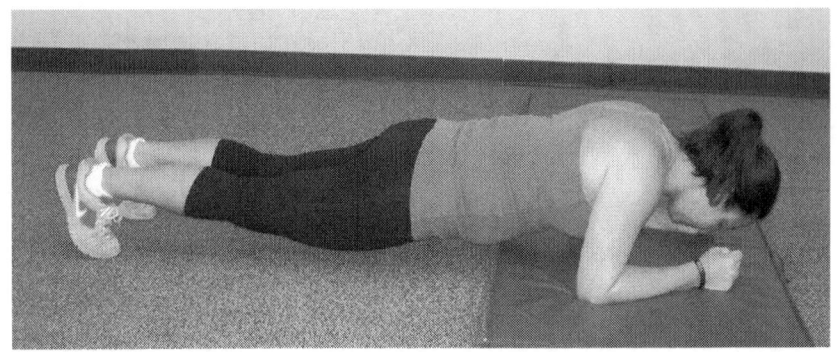

PITBP Bad Start – Elbows Misaligned Under Shoulders, Back is Hyperextended, Scapula Winged and Head is Misaligned with Shoulders

While maintaining good plank form, squeeze the glutes <u>HARD</u> until you feel a slight pelvic tilt take place. If you're having trouble picturing this in your mind's eye, think of making a fist with your butt. Hold for the required time, then release.

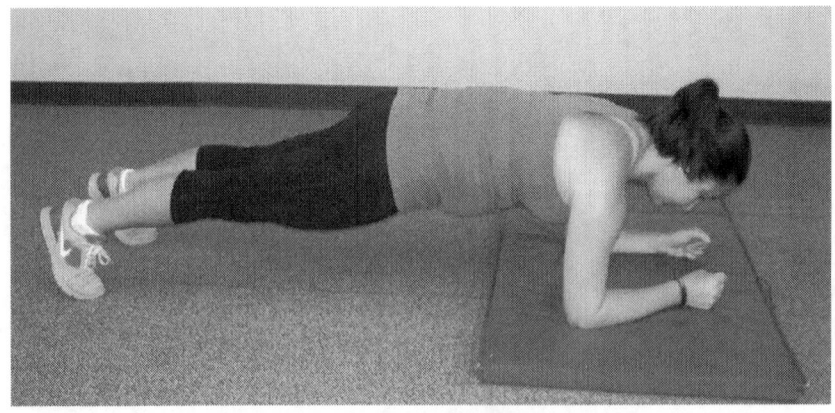

PITBP with Glutes Squeezed HARD!

Clapping Clam Shells (CCS)

Lie on your side with your feet drawn in so that your heels are about 8 to 10 inches from your butt. One leg should be resting atop the other. Imagine a straight line from your shoulder to your hip and then to your heels. Prop yourself up on your elbow and position the elbow directly under the shoulder.

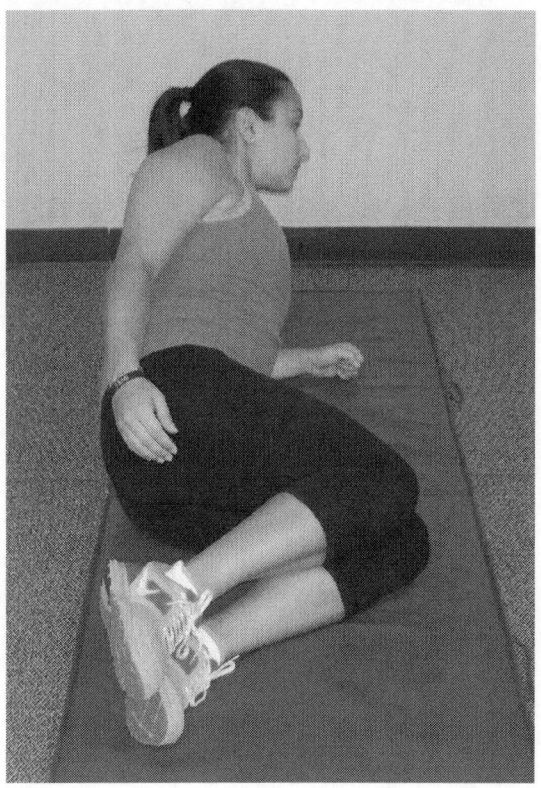

CCS Start – Straight Line From Shoulders to Ankles

Extend the free arm toward the ceiling while simultaneously driving through the knee of the leg on the ground. Raise the knee of the other leg so that it reaches for the ceiling and resembles a clam shell opening.

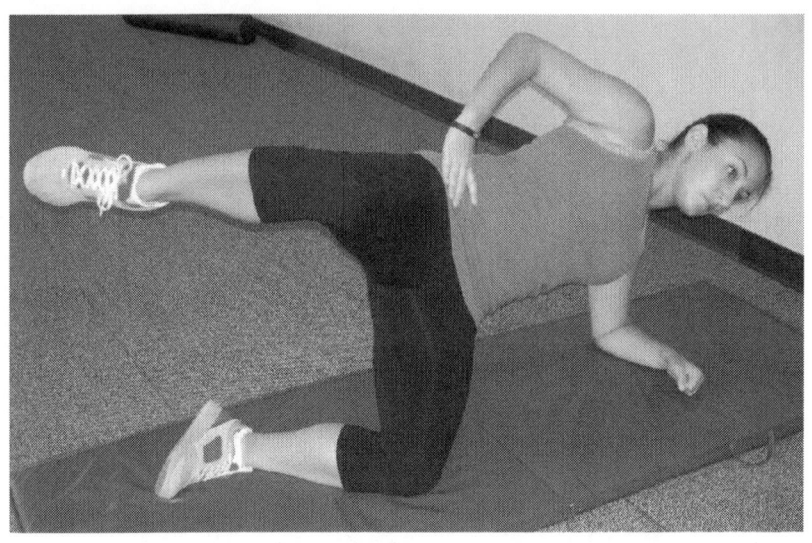

CCS Finish – Driving Through Grounded Knee and Extending Top Hip

Return under control and repeat.

Band Resisted Lateral Walks (BRLW)

Place the band across both legs. The further away from the knees the band is placed increases the difficulty of the exercise. So around the ankles or the arches of the feet is much tougher to do. Now, step out sideways so that you create a little resistance against the band. Lower your center of gravity by bending your knees. Keep the toes pointed straight ahead, or even slightly tilted inward (pigeon toed).

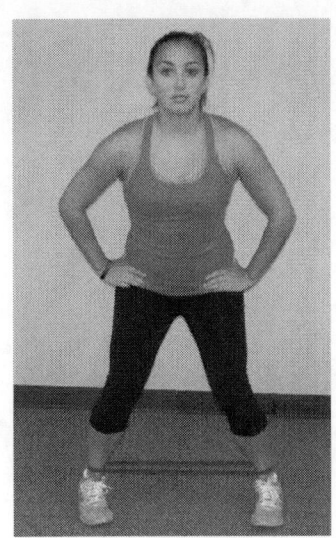

BRLW Start

Pick the foot up a couple of inches from the floor and step laterally about 10 to 15 inches. Plant that foot soundly, then do the same with the other foot. Do not let it drag across the floor, but rather pick it up and step.

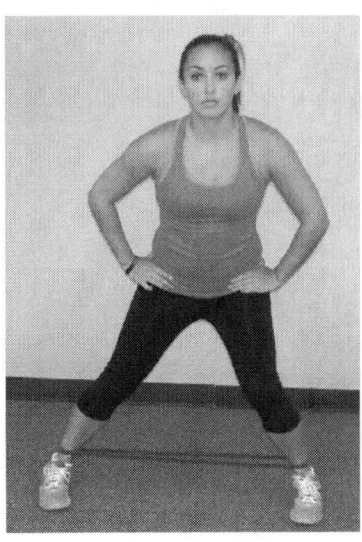

BRLW Finish Front View

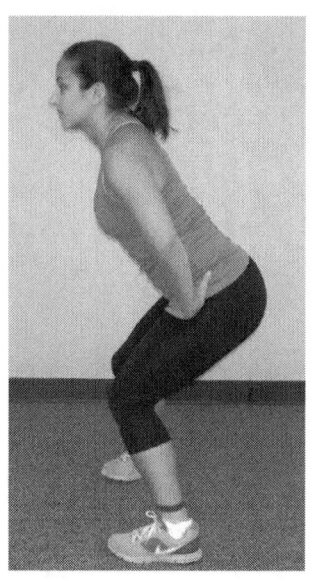

BRLW Side View

Do not allow the feet to get closer than hip width at any time during the exercise as this decreases the load and potential from the movement.

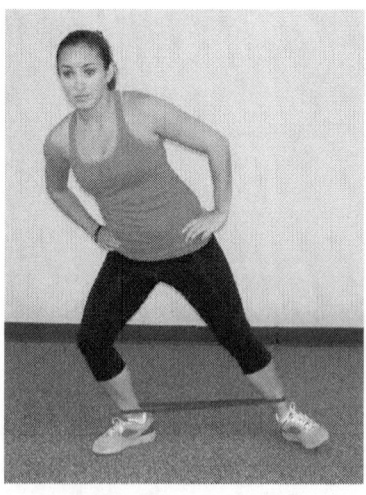

BRLW Bad Form – Leaning Upper Body, Toes Pointed Outward

Side Lying Hip Extensions (SLHE)

This one looks just like the Clapping Clam Shell exercise with the exception that the knees are in alignment with the hips, rather than extended forward.

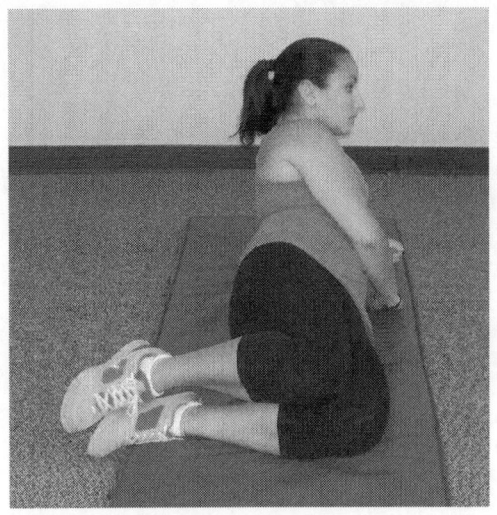

SLHE Start Side View

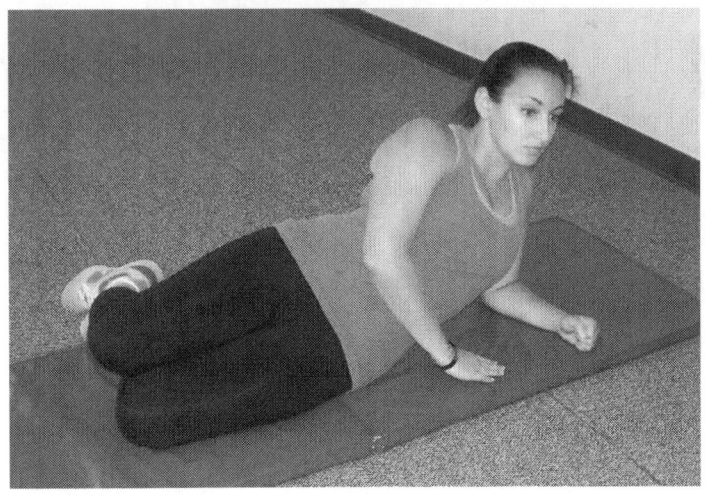

SLHE Start Front View

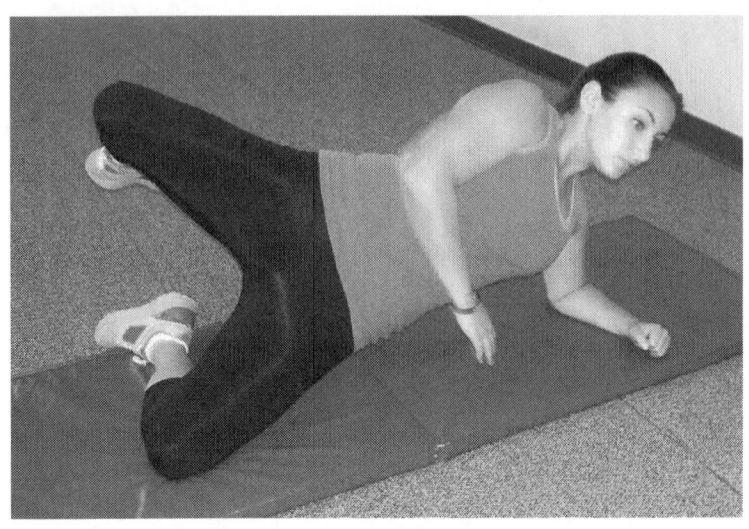

SLHE Finish

A Tighter Tummy AND Awesome Arms...In A Single Exercise?

Yes...it's true.

The plank, and its variations, which include the pushup, is that exercise. It's probably one of the most versatile movements on the planet, and can transform your body in no time.

Now, before you close the door on this idea, please here me out: they are not easy, but what in life truly worth having really is?

We earn the body in which we live, remember?

You can do this. Please let me tell you a quick story.

Hoover was one of the strongest men I've ever met, and he was 86 years old at the time.

I met him at a funeral near my home in San Antonio, Texas. The parents of a client had been killed in an auto accident, and I was attending their service. Afterward I was chatting with my client when Hoover approached we were introduced.

When I initially saw him, I knew he was not your typical 86 year old. He stood tall and straight, plus he had a grip like a vise.

I asked him, "Hoover, you are a very strong man. How do you do that?"

He simply smiled and stated, "I do 200 pushups every morning."

Hoover was apparently a fairly intuitive individual, and could sense my awe, probably because my jaw was now fully ajar. He knew before I could get it out where I was going with my next question, so he continued.

"Yep…I do 'em in sets of 20."

"You do 10 sets of 20 pushups each and every morning? How long have you been doing this?" I inquired.

He said, in a rather matter of fact tone, "I've been doing it for 50 years now."

I asked, "What else do you do? I mean for exercise?"

He smiled and said, "Does it look like I need to be doing anything else?"

More Than a Pushup

I hope you know that crunches and sit ups are NOT the best way to achieve a strong "core", or even a flat stomach, especially if you want keep your back healthy. No, a flat stomach is more a factor of diet. In the fitness industry we say, "Six pack abs are made in the kitchen."

Sit ups and crunches are just a good way to make your back hurt.

At my facility we never perform these things. They have no value to me and aren't worth the inherent risk. Rather we utilize the plank and its many variations. The pushup is nothing more than a moving plank. And most all of my clients have very strong core muscles. Do these properly and you will too.

You'll be utilizing 6 variations of the plank/push up combination over the next 31 days. Modify them as you need to by either elevating your upper body to a position where you can perform them well, or by doing them from your knees.

Here we go...

The Push Up and Reach (PU&R)

Begin by lying face down on the floor; your chin is tucked into the chest slightly so that your neck is in a neutral position. Your hands are in alignment with your pectoral muscles just outside the edge of your chest wall and your elbows are tucked in tight to your sides.

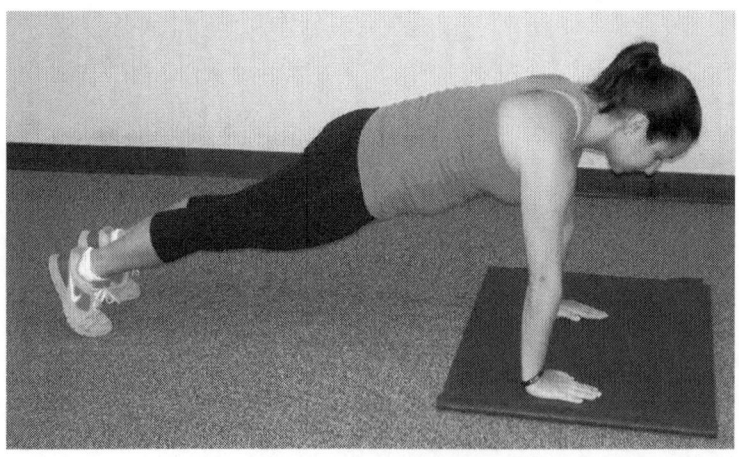

PU&R Initial Starting Position – Everything is TIGHT!

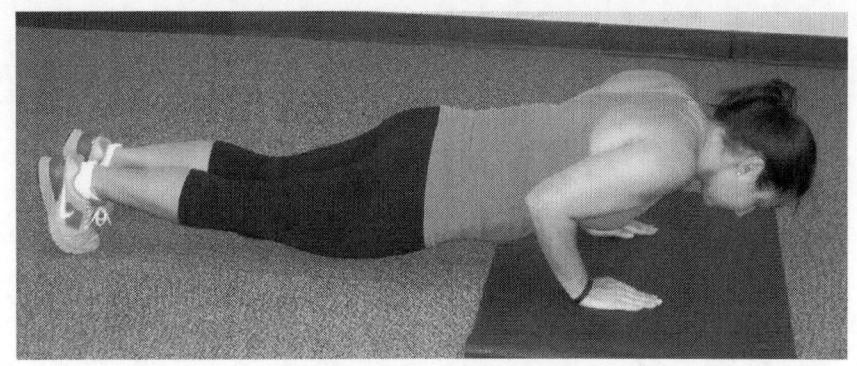

PU&R True Start Position

Squeeze your glutes and stomach region tightly, flex your thighs hard and exhale forcefully while pushing firmly through your palms into the floor. Keep pushing the floor away from you until your arms are completely locked out and your scapula (shoulder blades) are flat against the backside of your ribs. Your body should move seamlessly up, like a unit or plank of wood (now you know where that term comes from). When you reach the top of the movement, extend one arm in front of you while keeping the glutes, stomach, scapula and thighs squeezed tightly.

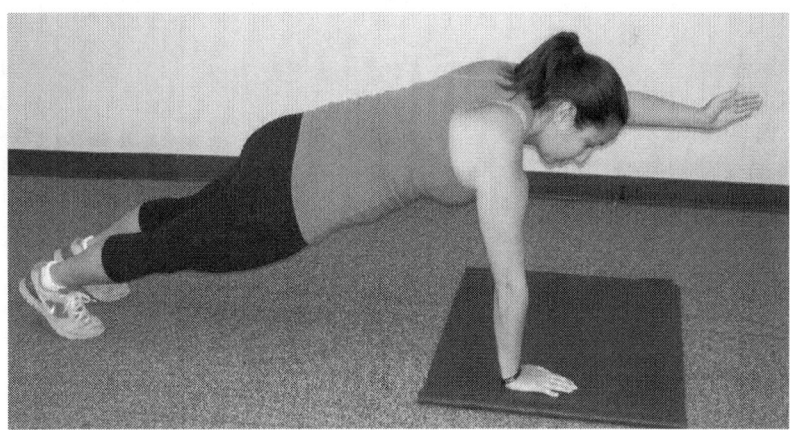

PU&R Finish Position

33

To reverse the motion, place your hand back onto the ground, keep your body tightly aligned in that plank position and inhale gently, then… **and this is the key!!**… bend your elbows before your shoulder blades collapse. Now, under control, slowly lower yourself to the floor until your chest just touches the floor. Do not rest on the floor but keep tension through the body and repeat.

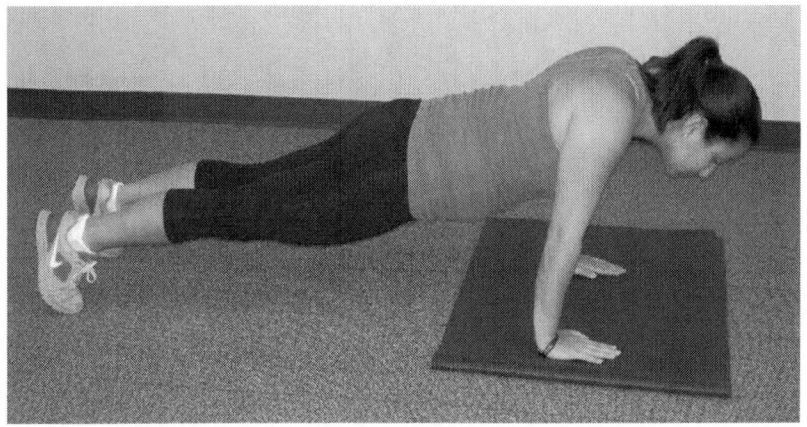

PU&R Bad Initial Start Position – Shoulders Have Caved in BEFORE the Elbows Have Begun to Bend, Head and Chin Have Drifted Forward

It is extremely important that the tension between your shoulder blades remains taut so that your shoulder capsule is not compromised before your pectoral muscles and triceps take over. Practice this movement at an inclined level like a counter top or back of the couch if you cannot maintain good form at floor level during the exercise.

Atomic Plank And Push Up (AP&PU)

Start in the forward plank position. Keeping the stomach and glutes tight, using your arms rise from the plank position to the push up start position, perform a complete push up, then lower yourself back into the forward plank position. This constitutes one repetition.

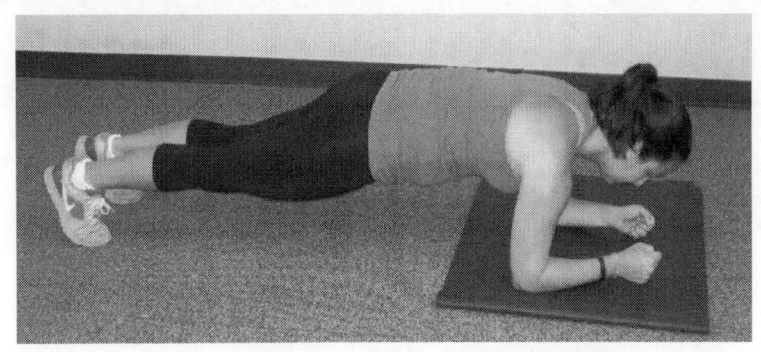

AP&PU Start Position (Planking Phase)

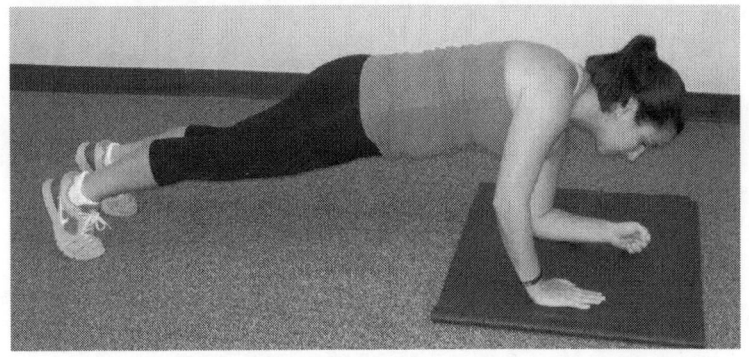

AP&PU Intermediate Position (Transition Phase)

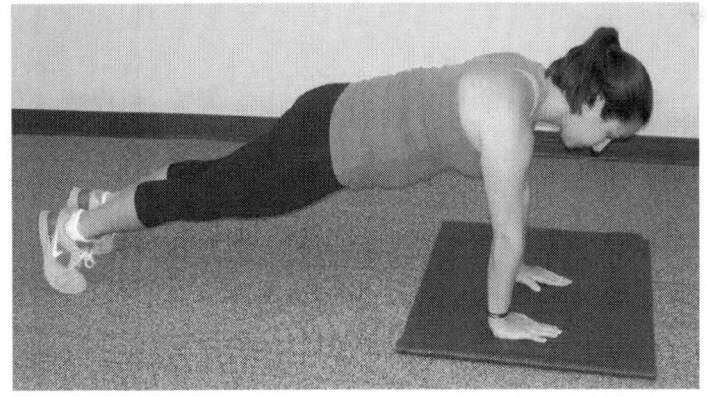

AP&PU Top Position (Start of Push Up Phase)

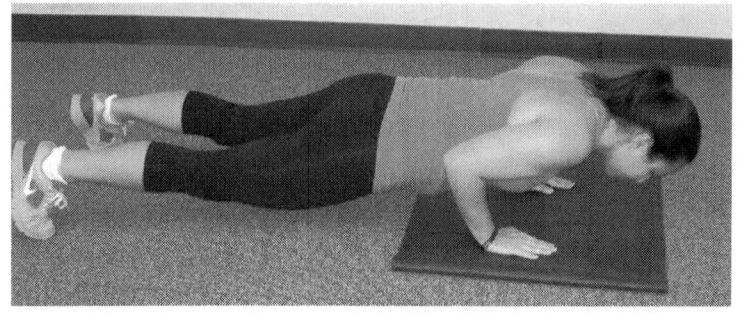

AP&PU Bottom Position (End of Push Up Phase)

Be sure to stay tight throughout the exercise and do not allow the hips to rise (mountain top) or buckle (valley) excessively.

Side Plank and Rotating Reach (SPRR)

Lie on the ground on your side with the elbow of one arm on the floor directly under the shoulder. Squeeze your stomach tight, squeeze your glutes tight so that there is a straight line from your shoulders to ankles and raise your hips from the floor. Keep your chin tucked slightly and do not allow your head to tilt downward toward the floor. Raise your other arm upward and slightly back, as if reaching for a wall.

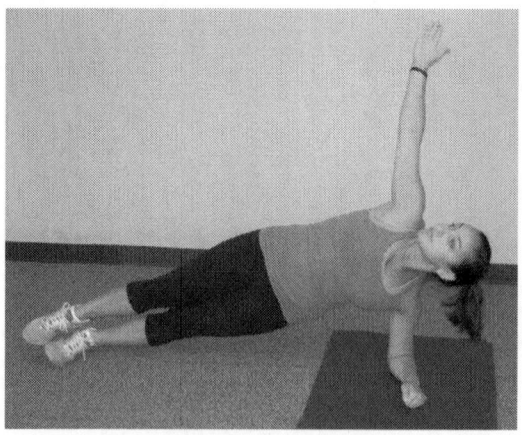

SPRR Start Position

Inhale gently and roll your chest toward the floor while sweeping your arm underneath your body and extend your hand as if reaching for the wall behind you. Do your best to keep your hips tight and a straight line from shoulders to ankles.

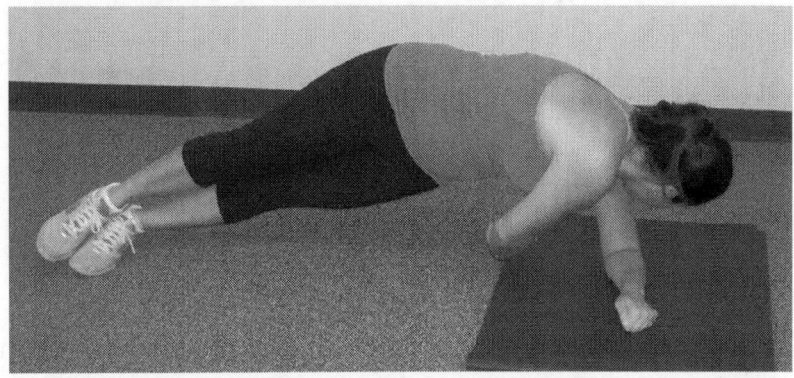

SPRR Finish Position

Exhale as you roll under control back into the starting position, keeping everything nice and tight.

Push Up and Pike (PU&P)

You will need something upon which to place your feet that slides. Depending upon what type of flooring you have (hard like tile or wood, soft like carpet) you can use anything that will slide across the floor.

For carpeted floors I use a flexible cutting board, which you can find at Bed, Bath & Beyond for about $6. They'll last for years and slide very easily on carpet. A slick magazine cover, piece of cardboard or even an old X-ray exposure works well too.

For hard floors, a 12x12 piece of old shag carpet works pretty well.

Begin in the proper push up position with your feet on the sliding piece. Do a push up under control and with great form and technique.

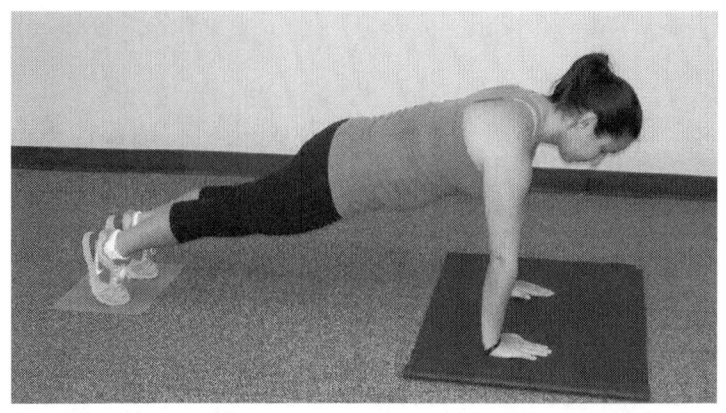

PU&P Start Position of Both Push Up and Pike

Once you return to the arms locked out, start position of the push up, contract your stomach muscles and draw your hips skyward as high as you can. Return to the push up position under control.

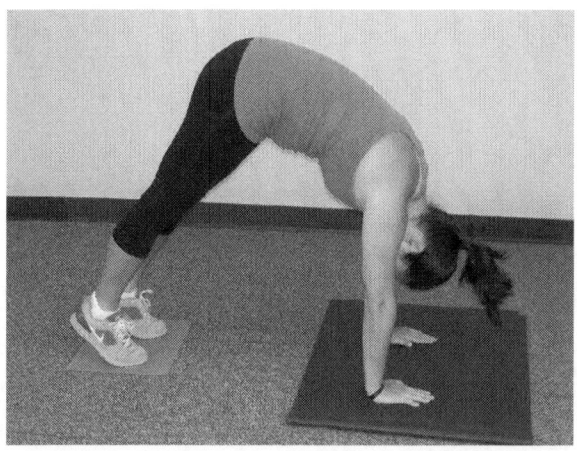

PU&P Finish Position Knees Locked With Hips High

If this maneuver is too difficult, you can just draw your knees into your chest while keeping your hips as parallel to the floor as possible. Return to the push up position under control to begin the next repetition.

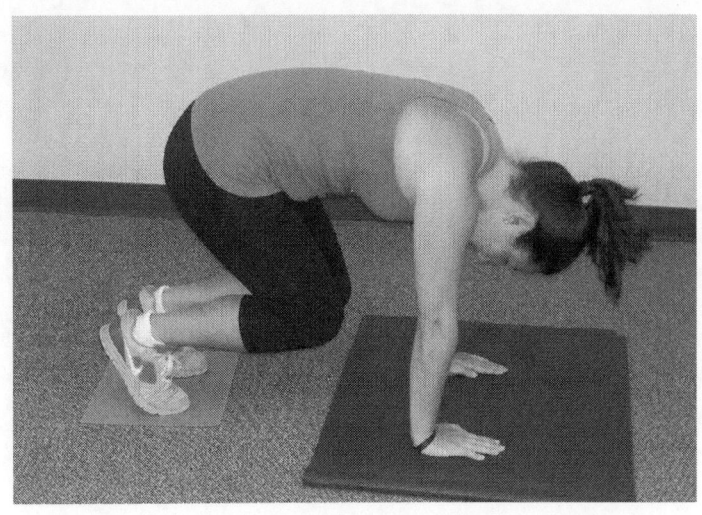

PU&P Position Finish With Knees Bent and Hips Low

The Saw (SAW)

You will once again need the sliding piece from the Pike exercise above.

Get into the forward plank position with your elbows directly under your shoulders and your toes on the slide. Squeeze your stomach and glutes **HARD** and raise your hips into the proper planked position.

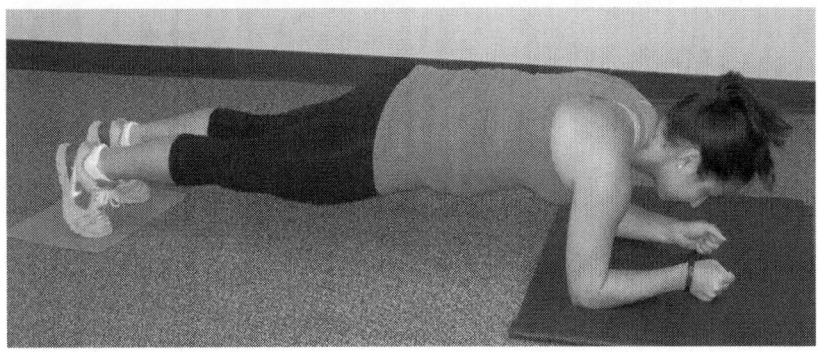

SAW Start – Good Plank With Elbows Directly Under Shoulders

Keeping your body in the rigid plank position with your glutes squeezed very tightly, move from your elbows backward, sliding your feet across the floor as you move.

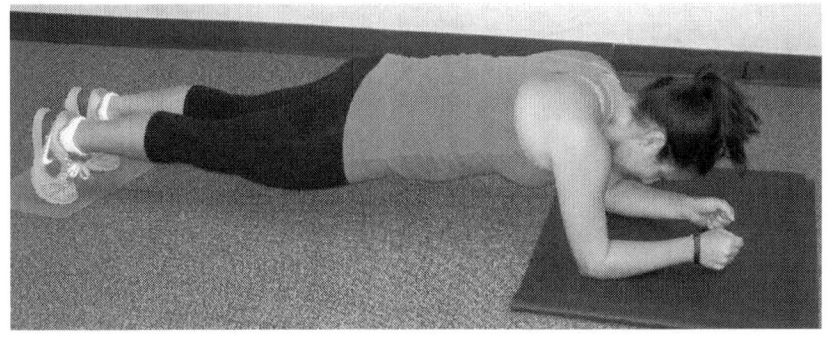

SAW Finish – Good Plank, Body Extended Backward Moving Only at the Shoulders, Glutes and Shoulders Tight

Be careful not to move more than a couple of inches at first, in order to gauge how well you respond to this most difficult movement. If you feel any pain or pinching in the low back, do one of two things:

1. Minimize your range of motion so as to move in a pain free manner, or
2. Step off of the slide and simply dorsiflex and plantarflex (bend the ankles forward and backward) the ankles.

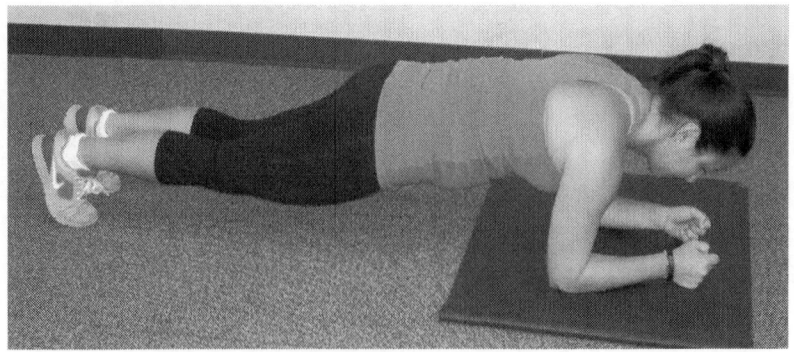

SAW Start With No Slide – Ankles Dorsiflexed

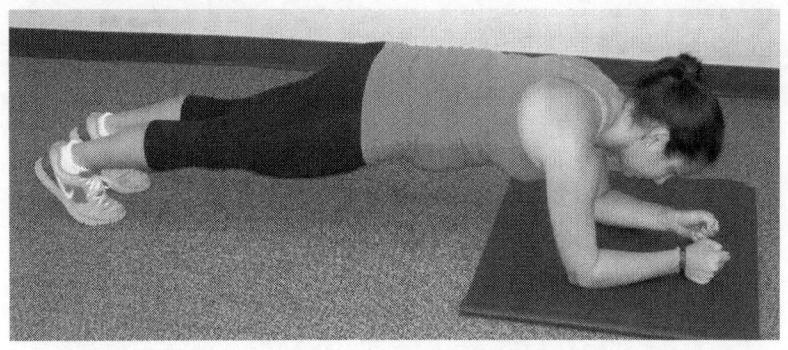

SAW Finish With No Slide – Ankles Plantarflexed

If you still have trouble doing this one without pain, eliminate it from the routine, substitute it for another of these exercises and get yourself checked out by a professional to find out why it is you hurt.

Push Up and 180 Degree Spin (PU&180)

The final exercise is going to require you to think a little while you move.

Begin in good push up form and perform a quality push up, then while you maintain strict push up form (as best you can) rotate 180 degrees and position yourself into proper push up position once again.

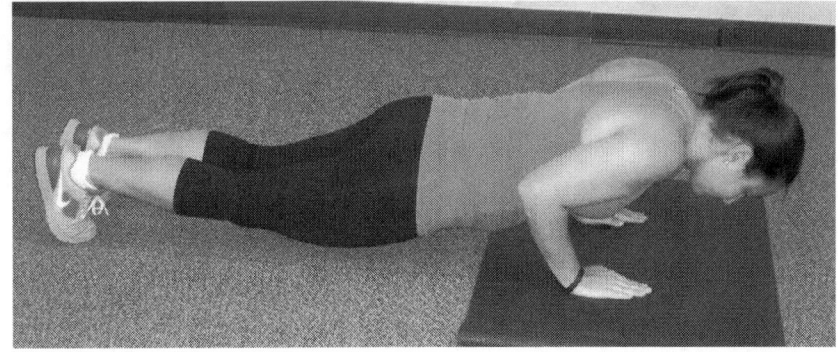

PU&180 Start Phase

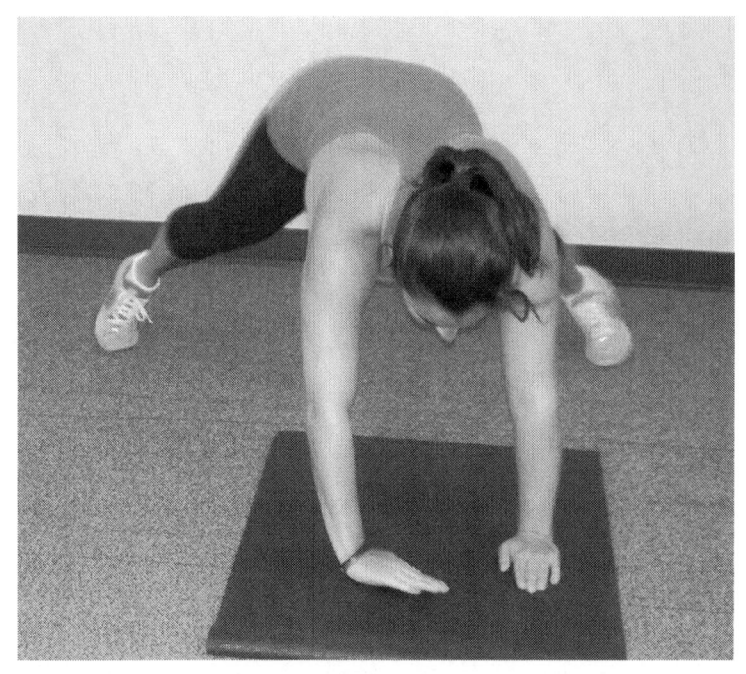

PU&180 Transition Phase

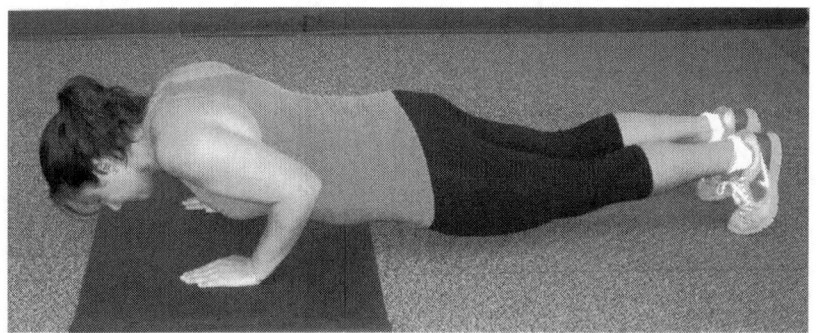

PU&180 Restart Phase

Perform another push up and then spin another 180 degrees for the required number of repetitions.

These are the exercises you will be performing for the next 31 days. In conjunction with good eating, and the 31 day program I'm about to lay out for you, you should see significant changes to your strength, shape and capability in that time.

The 31 Day Program

Follow this plan to the best of your capability. Rest and/or take breaks as you need to, especially if your form and technique are getting compromised. But do not quit.

You'll train for 6 days, and then take a day off. Each training session can be completed in under 30-40 minutes easily if you minimize your rest.

Be sure to warm up thoroughly before each day's training session.

Be mindful and focus on what you're doing and use good form and technique on each and every exercise to get most from these 31 days.

Drink plenty of pure water before, during and after.

Eat a quality, supportive, whole food, single ingredient meal plan each and every day and you'll be amazed at what you accomplish.

I promise.

If you will dedicate yourself to this program, not compromising with lame excuses or "cop outs", you will be amazed at what you will accomplish and learn about yourself.

You're stronger than you think you are.

I know it.

Do you?

Here we go…

1	2	3	4	5	6	7
100 Squat 30 Single Leg RDL 15 Push Up & Reach	100 Shoulder Elevated Hip Lift 30 Lying Band Resisted Hip Drive 15 Atomic Plank & Push UP	50 Reverse Lunges 3 X 20 Count Pain in the Butt Plank 15 Push Up & Pike	50 Single Leg Shoulders Elevated Hip Lift 20 Clapping Clam Shells 10 Saw	40 Rear Foot Elevated Split Squats 40 Band Resisted Lateral Walks 15 Side Plank Reach & Rotate	50 Hips Elevated Walk Outs 20 Side Lying Hip Extensions Push Ups and a 180 Degree Spin X 15	REST

8	9	10	11	12	13	14
150 Squat 40 SLRDL 20 PU&R	150 SEHL 40 LBRHD 20 AP&PU	60 RL 2X30 Ct PITBP 20 PU&P	70 SLSEHL 30 CCS 15 SAW	50 RFESS 60 BRLW 20 SPR&R	75 HEWO 25 SLHE PU&180 X 20	REST

15	16	17	18	19	20	21
200 Squat	200 SEHL	70 RL	90 SLSEHL	60 RFESS	100 HEWO	REST
50 SLRDL	50 LBRHD	3X30 Ct PITBP	40 CCS	80 BRLW	30 SLHE	
25 PU&R	25 AP&PU	25 PU&P	20 SAW	25 SPR&R	PU&180 X 25	

22	23	24	25	26	27	28
250 Squat	250 SEHL	90 RL	100 SLHEHL	70 RFESS	125 HEWO	REST
60 SLRDL	60 LBRHD	4X30 Ct PITBP	50 CCS	100 BRLW	40 SLHE	
30 PU&R	30 AP&PU	30 PU&P	25 SAW	30 SPR&R	PU&180 X 30	

22	23	24	25	26	27	28
250 Squat	250 SEHL	90 RL	100 SLHEHL	70 RFESS	125 HEWO	REST
60 SLRDL	60 LBRHD	4X30 Ct PITBP	50 CCS	100 BRLW	40 SLHE	
30 PU&R	30 AP&PU	30 PU&P	25 SAW	30 SPR&R	PU&180 X 30	

29	30	31
300 Squat	300 SEHL	100 RL
75 SLRDL	75 LBRHD	2X45 Ct PITBP
40 PU&R	40 AP&PU	40 PU&P

There you have it. The outcome is up to you.

If you have any questions, or if I can be of service to you in some way, please contact me: Steve@firestormfitcamps.com

Also please go to www.firestormfitcamps.com and sign up for my free newsletter and when you do you'll have the opportunity to download up to 20 FREE reports on virtually every aspect of fitness success.

And I promise, we'll never spam you or give your info away because that just sucks...

About Steve Payne

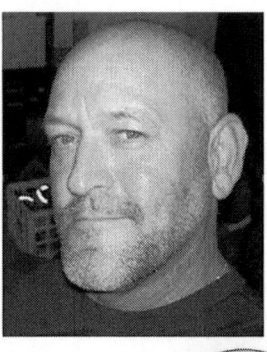

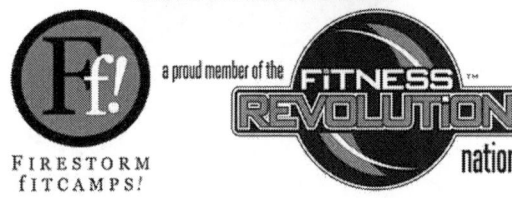

Steve Payne is a 30+ year veteran of the health, fitness and sports performance industry and has trained over two thousand people in that time.

He is the owner of Firestorm fitcamps! as well as a proud franchise member of the Fitness Revolution Nation. Steve is a husband of 15 years to Kennon Marie, father to Kristina and Stephanie and grandfather to Christian Scott, Conner Nicolaus, Jozef Devin and Hunter Steven. Steve is a cat lover and he and Kennon enjoy and live with 7 cats: Bella, Bunny, BB, Bizette, Scruffy (the one-eyed wonder), KC and Katniss.

www.firestormfitcamps.com
facebook.com/FirestormfitcampsSA

www.aminuteofpayne.com
https://www.facebook.com/AMinuteOfPayne

CHAPTER 2

Igor Klibanov

It's Not Your Fault You're Fat, It's Your Hormones-How to Eat Wisely, Take Control of Your Hormones & Lose Weight Naturally

"Estrogen should be a controlled substance", one speaker said at a motivational talk. Granted, the gentleman lives in a home with a wife and two daughters (whom he loves very much).

At one of the most popular talks that I give, titled "7 Dangerous Facts That Will Backfire and Cause You to Stay Fat or Hurt Yourself", I always make a point of educating the audience that your hormones influence your body fat far more than calories. Yes, calories still matter, but they are an afterthought.

Want proof?

Take a type 1 diabetic. If that person eats 10,000 calories per day, but doesn't inject insulin, he will lose weight.

Or on the opposite end of the spectrum, and what so many frustrated clients come to me with: thyroid problems. People who have poor thyroid function can eat as few as 1200 calories per day (that's well below the starvation line), and still gain body fat.

What you (just as many of my fat loss clients) may not know is that you may have an underactive thyroid, even if your blood work says that you're "normal."

In this chapter, we'll discuss how and why hormones can influence fat loss, as well as how to train, eat and supplement for the balance of different hormones.

What Causes Hormonal Imbalances?

I feel like before answering this question, I need to give a disclaimer. I am not a doctor. I am a fitness author (I wrote two books, called *STOP EXERCISING! The Way You Are Doing it Now. 7 Dangerous Facts That Will Backfire and Cause You to Stay Fat or Hurt Yourself* as well as *Unlimited Progress: How You Can Unlock Your Body's Potential*), a speaker, and a fitness professional. But not a doctor.

I know about restoring balance when it is not a true pathology. I help people handle that zone when you're doctor says that you're healthy, but you know that you don't feel healthy.

I also know about restoring balance only as it pertains to fat loss or muscle gain/toning (though if you'd like some professional help with that, check out the FREE gift at the end of this chapter. With that out of the way, let's answer the question "what causes hormonal imbalances?"

Hormone imbalances don't just "happen", and they certainly don't appear as a simple result of aging. Sure, aging will increase some hormones and decrease others, but you should gracefully go from youth into old age without a plethora of symptoms. So what's the cause?

Many times, hormonal imbalances can be traced back to two or three root causes:

1. Stress
2. Poor health of the digestive system

50

3. Poor thyroid function

The implication of this is simple. Fix the above factors, and very often, other problems that seem unrelated either go away entirely, or improve tremendously.

How Does Stress Cause Hormonal Imbalances?

First of all, let's clear up a misconception. Stress isn't just mental/emotional (like relationships, finances, deadlines, etc.). Stress refers to a lot of other things, like:

- Poor nutrition
- Dehydration
- Poor sleep
- Prescription medications
- Pollution
- Radiation
- And more

The effect on your hormones is still the same: fluctuations and imbalances. When stress increases, so does the hormone cortisol. And that's the way it should be, since cortisol is a helpful hormone in times of stress that helps mobilize fuel for an emergency.

So sugar is released into the blood. But wait. You're just sitting there. Unlike your ancient ancestors, who ran away when they felt stress (after all, the only form of stress in the ancient world was a sabre toothed tiger chasing you), you're sitting at your desk and fuming. That blood sugar doesn't go into muscle, but stays in your blood. So to bring down your blood sugar, you need to release insulin.

But stress doesn't just play around with cortisol and insulin. It also depletes a "brain chemical" called "serotonin." If you have less serotonin, you don't feel as good. You self-medicate with "treats" like sugar, pastries, etc.

51

Stress also makes your body less sensitive to a hormone called "leptin." Leptin is a hormone released by your fat cells that tells your brain that you're full. So you might still have leptin floating around in your blood, but your brain just doesn't "hear" the message.

Let's not forget estrogen and progesterone. Under times of stress, your body doesn't want to make babies. It just wants to survive. So your estrogen is decreased, as is your progesterone.

All this adds up to you not just having a few bulges here and there, but all these hormonal imbalances can lead to:

- Sugar cravings
- Salt cravings
- Bags under your eyes
- Problems with your periods
- Decreased sex drive
- Fatigue
- Coffee cravings
- Feeling cold all the time, even when others around you are quite comfortable
- Forgetfulness
- Anxiety
- Depression
- And more

So how do we manage stress? Although I am a fitness professional, I like to give my clients the complete package: exercise, nutrition, supplementation, and lifestyle.

So in terms of exercise, you want to do what helps you relieve stress. The worst exercise you can do for a stressed-out body is excessive cardiovascular activity. Any "cardio" increases the stress hormones in your body.

Not exactly what you need, considering there's already too much of them in your body. So opt for more gentle activities, like yoga, walking, gentle stretching, etc. This isn't a "forever" type of recommendation.

This is just until your hormones are back in balance (which can take 1 month – 2 years or more), after which point, you can use more "traditional" fat loss training (a combination of strength training and cardio). In the meantime, you'll actually lose more body fat with the gentle approach than with the hardcore approach. If you're wondering about how to exercise properly, it's covered in my free home study course at
http://fatlossforwomencourse.com.

As far as nutrition is concerned, the keys are to eliminate or replace the biggest stressors on your body: refined foods. Things like sugar, pastries, white bread, and white pasta can be replaced with more healthful options.

I know that if you've been doing some independent health "research", you're wondering "what about potatoes and carrots?" I wouldn't worry about that too much. Continue eating those foods, just replace anything that is processed or refined. Those tend to be the biggest stressors on the body. No calorie counting required.

As far as supplementation is concerned, besides a high-quality multi-vitamin (if you want to figure out what's "high quality", check out this article: www.torontofitnessonline.com/nutritional-supplement/), you should supplement with vitamin C, B complex, and vitamin B5 (you usually need more than what's found in your multi-vitamin and the B-complex). Why those specific nutrients? Those are the ones depleted the most when a person is under stress.

And lifestyle. Often the toughest part. You see, stress is often about perception. What's stressful to one person may be delightful to another person. So perception plays a big role. Sleep is also critical towards helping you balance your hormones.

Do everything in your power to get the sleep you need, and manage your stress. There are plenty of stress management strategies that are effective.

With one of my clients, a 46-year-old mother of two, my "prescription" was very short workouts (about 30 minutes), 10-12 hours of sleep per day (can be broken up), a multi-vitamin, vitamin C, B complex, B5, and a number of herbs specific to her stress profile (different people experience stress differently. Some people are wired, others are tired, others are cold, others catch colds, etc.

There are 6 different stress profiles, and different herbs are helpful for different profiles). Over the next 3 months, she was able to drop 9 pounds of body fat, while gaining 8 pounds of muscle. She shrunk 2 dress sizes, and started wearing a dress with an open back to her dancing classes, something she was too embarrassed to do before.

How Does Digestion Affect Fat Loss?

The digestive system is a long tube, and a lot of different things can go wrong. But two of the most common are insufficient stomach acid and insufficient enzymes.

Stomach acid is necessary to break down protein, and absorb a number of nutrients (like calcium, zinc, B12, iron, and others). So if you don't have enough stomach acid, it's a recipe for problems with fat loss.

Plus, problems in the northern part of the digestive system will affect everything south of them. The stomach is north of the small intestine and large intestine.

How do we develop insufficient stomach acid? There are a number of ways, but chief among them are excessive stress, and the deficiencies of certain nutrients (especially zinc and vitamin B1).

To restore stomach acid, first find out how deficient you are. To do that, you'll need to perform the betaine HCl challenge test (just Google it), and then begin the corrective program.

The other major issue is insufficient enzymes. Enzymes are found primarily in the small intestine, and they help break down things like fats and carbohydrates. If you're deficient in enzymes, your fats and carbs don't get broken down, and the result can be gas, bloating, and yes, fat loss resistance.

To correct enzyme deficiency, the first order of business is to fix your stomach acid. Remember, everything north in the digestive system affects everything south. Assuming your stomach acid is sufficient, it's not a bad idea to supplement with digestive enzymes, until your body naturally starts producing them.

The Thyroid Connection

The thyroid is a butterfly-shaped gland sitting in the middle of your throat, and it's the "gas pedal" on your metabolism. When the thyroid starts to malfunction, your metabolism slows down, so no matter how well you eat or how much you exercise, you'll still be predisposed to fat gain. Here are some signs that may indicate slow thyroid function:

- Difficulty losing weight even with a low calorie intake
- Feeling cold in your hands and feet, even when others around you are comfortable
- Low energy
- Low libido
- Thinning hair on the outer third of your eyebrow.
- Low tolerance for exercise (you get tired quickly)
- Anemia

Want a pretty close to surefire way to figure out whether your thyroid is malfunctioning? Measure your body temperature in the armpit (not in the mouth or ear or um… other cavities) for 10 minutes.

This should be done before even getting out of bed first thing in the morning. Your temperature should be 36.5-36.8 Celsius (that's 97.8-98.2 Fahrenheit). If it's less than 36.5 degrees, your metabolism is slow.

For every degree Celsius that you're under this range, your metabolism is 20% slower. So if your temperature is 35.5-35.8, you're burning 20% less calories per day than you should be. If your temperature is 34.5-34.8, you're burning 40% fewer calories per day than you should be.

Whenever a new client starts working with me, with the goal of fat loss, I notice that in more than 90% of cases, they have low body temperature.

The implication of this is quite simple: raise your body temperature to what's optimal, and your metabolism is restored. Once your metabolism is back, firing on all cylinders, fat loss becomes much easier.

How do we get your metabolism back on track? An approach that I learned from Matt Stone , (owner of 180degreeheadlth.com),
is we do the exact opposite of what you did to slow it down: eat more and exercise less. What? Yes, read that again: eat more and exercise less. Did you ever think that a fitness professional would ever tell you to do those things?

The primary cause of the metabolism slowing down is yo-yo dieting. You see, your body can't tell the difference between a diet and a famine.

So when you go on a diet, your body thinks there's a famine going on, so to protect you against future "famines", it slows down your metabolism. This way you burn fewer calories, which makes you more likely to survive the next "famine." Great for survival. Not so great for health and looking good.

To get your body to go in the other direction, you'll need to eat until you're slightly uncomfortably full. Yes, you'll gain some body fat during this time (although it won't be as much as you think), but you'll speed up your metabolism in the process.

This way, once you resume normal eating, you'll burn body fat without really trying. It will just be a side effect of your metabolism firing on all cylinders. Think of it as taking one step back to take two steps forward.

56

Oh, and the biggest benefit of all? You will not regain the weight that you lost.

Now, just a word of caution. When women gain fat while they're restoring their metabolism, they freak out, and go on another diet. And they're back in the vicious cycle. Don't let that be you. It's important to continue eating until your temperature returns to 36.5-36.8.

At that point, you can go back to moderation. And yes, it can be a very emotional experience when your favorite clothes start feeling tight, so it may not be a bad idea to be held accountable by a professional or a friend/family member.

That's just the eating side of things.
Why do you want to avoid exercise at this time? Because contrary to what you've been told, exercise doesn't speed up the metabolism. It slows it down.

Especially endurance exercise (that includes jogging, swimming, cycling, etc.). Moderate amounts of strength training and certainly stretching don't seem to have this effect, but endurance training does.

So keep your exercise very light (things like light walking, tai chi, gentle stretching, etc. all fit the bill. Or if you feel like just doing nothing at this time, that's fine too). Again, this is just temporary, until your metabolism has been restored.

Now, let's talk supplementation. Besides a high-quality multi-vitamin, it's not a bad idea to take a thyroid-support supplement. While I don't endorse any particular company, a good supplement will at the very least contain:

L-Tyrosine
Iodine
Selenium

It may very well contain other ingredients, but just make sure that it has these basic 3.

Fix Your Other Hormones

Now that you've taken care of your stress levels, improved your digestive health, and optimized thyroid function, you're in much better shape, and much more primed for fat loss. However, if you still have a few lingering symptoms (and many of you will not) even after 2-3 months of fixing all of the above, it's time to fix your other hormones. Fortunately, it'll be much easier to fix them now, rather than before addressing your stress, digestion and thyroid.

Hopefully by now you understand that a prerequisite to fat loss is hormonal balance. If there is no hormonal balance, you can forget about fat loss. Yes, you might lose it for a short while, but it'll come back (and often, you'll gain more than you lost).

The nice thing is that once your hormones are restored, fat loss is a side effect. It just happens, without any real conscious effort on your part. You'll naturally feel like exercising, and crave foods that are healthy for you. It won't be a constant struggle.

FREE GIFT - 1

Special Opportunity for Readers of "Bodyweight Exercises for Women"

The Most Incredible FREE Gift Ever
($319 Worth of Pure Body-Changing, Performance-Enhancing Information)

Igor Klibanov is offering an incredible opportunity for you to see WHY Fitness Solutions Plus is known as "THE Go-To COMPANY" where mature, confident women seeking EFFECTIVE and Sustainable Fat Loss and greater Energy go.

Igor wants to give you $319 worth of pure Body-Changing, Energy-Increasing information including a personalized Dream Body MAP

Session, Biosignature Assessment, and a Myoneural Injury Risk Trigenics Assessment. You'll receive a complete map of your body.

Dream Body MAP Session

- How <u>any</u> woman can lose body fat without starvation or calorie counting
- **How to avoid exercise and nutrition programs that don't work**
- How you can fit into your favourite clothes
- **The BIGGEST MISTAKE most women make in their training and nutrition**

Biosignature Assessment: The ESSENTIALS Towards Optimizing Body Composition

- How to optimize your body fat and lean muscle mass to look and feel your best
- **Key elements that determine your body fat (it's not just calories)**
- How to lose body fat the right way <u>for you</u>
- **Which food and supplements you should use to tighten and tone your body.**

Myoneural Injury Risk Trigenics Assessment

- How to INSTANTLY improve strength by working on your muscle-nerve connection
- **How to quickly increase your range of motion** without long-duration static stretching
- How to prevent an injury before it happens
- **How to decrease constant tightness in your neck, back or legs.**
-

These FREE Gifts are redeemed at our facility in Markham, Ontario, Canada (5 minutes north of Toronto).

To redeem them, visit
www.torontofitnessonline.com/dream-body-map-session

FREE GIFT - 2

Fat Loss for the Mature, Confident Woman

In this home study course, you'll learn:

- Why women gain body fat during perimenopause and menopause
- How to eat right at that time in your life
- How to de-stress to lose weight
- What is the right way to exercise at that point in your life
- What supplements are helpful

You can get it by going to www.FatLossForWomenCourse.com.

About Igor Klibanov

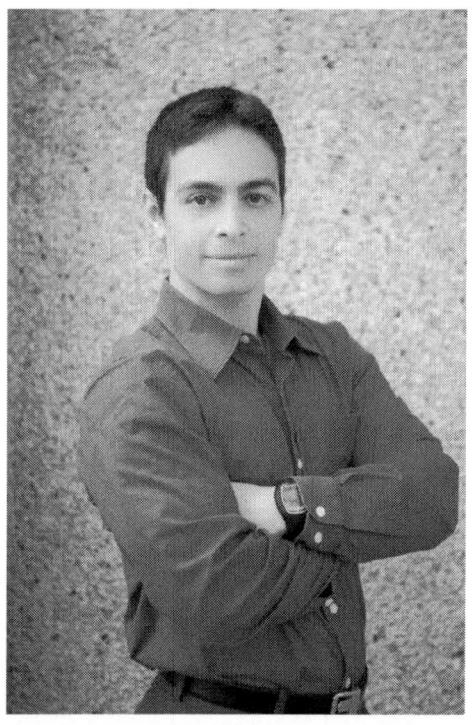

Igor Klibanov was selected as one of the top 5 personal trainers in Toronto by the Metro News newspaper on June 3, 2010. He is the founder and owner of Fitness Solutions Plus, a personal training and fitness/health education company.

Igor began training in martial arts at a young age, and enjoyed learning about movement and the human body enough to pursue a degree in kinesiology and health science from York University.

Graduating in 2009, he worked as a personal trainer for a country club and community centre, before founding Fitness Solutions Plus in early 2010.

Currently, only 2 years since founding Fitness Solutions Plus, he has been able to train a number of local TV personalities, CEOs of well-known organizations, and delivered fitness education seminars at many well-known companies, including Investors Group, Sunlife, and Soberman LLC.

Igor strongly believes in continued education, and at the time of this writing (in June 2013) has the following qualifications:

- B.A. (Specialized Honours) kinesiology and health science
- Biosignature Practitioner
- Certified Trigenics Trainer (CTT)
- Canadian Society of Exercise Physiology (CSEP) Certified Personal Trainer (CPT)
- Can-Fit-Pro Personal Trainer Specialist (PTS)

Igor has a free fitness newsletter. You can subscribe to it by simply visiting his website at www.TorontoFitnessOnline.com

Igor would be glad to hear what you think of this book, so please don't hesitate to email him at
Igor@TorontoFitnessOnline.com

To book Igor as a speaker at your event, please email him at
Igor@TorontoFitnessOnline.com.

CHAPTER 3

Nicole LaBonde

How to Love Bodyweight Exercises & Your Bodyweight Exercise Checklist

Strength training often gets neglected by women. We know we *should* do it. But we don't. There is a fear of "bulking up", of hurting ourselves, of looking foolish trying to figure out what the machine actually *does*! But I'm here to tell you- strength training is KEY to your overall fitness.

This goes beyond looking good in a strapless dress or mini skirt. (Although, that's great, and I'm going to give you access for a free bonus that targets those areas!) Strength training has lifelong effects on your entire body.

More muscle means less fat. More muscle means your body will continue to burn calories long after your workout is finished. And, when done properly, more muscle actually means more flexibility, not bulk!

In the rest of this chapter I'm going to give you:
- 5 reasons to LOVE bodyweight exercises

- 3 things to keep in mind when performing your bodyweight exercies
- 5 great bodyweight exercises that use resistance to create strength in the target area, AND the whole body

What to LOVE About Bodyweight Exercises:

1. **We get the most out of our bodyweight exercises when we perform them with resistance.**
   This means fighting gravity. The way to think of it is: "use your muscles, not your joints". When we use resistance, we use our muscles in two ways- to perform the movement AND to resist it. This is like a double workout! Resistance is the key to proper execution of bodyweight exercises.

   If you hate lunges because your knees fatigue before your quads do, or you feel like you can't get enough arm work with bodyweight exercise, this chapter is for YOU! I'm going to give you some examples and coaching that will have you feeling your thighs and triceps in no time!

2. **Proper execution of bodyweight exercises will lead not just to stronger target muscles, but also increased flexibility.**

   In these exercises we're performing with resistance, our muscle engagement is equal in both contraction AND extension. This is what makes the long, lean lines of so many dancers and Pilates instructors. You are stretching and strengthening, at the same time! A muscle has to be strong in order to stretch, so your joints are supported. A muscle also needs flexibility to increase strength, or your range of motion will be limited.

3. **Bodyweight exercises also increases strength in your small, internal postural muscles.**

Those muscles are constantly firing when bodyweight exercises are done properly. And they are especially important as we age. They help hold us upright, control our movements, and increase our fine motor skills.

Strength in these muscles leads to internal stability, which in turn, increases our balance and coordination. These postural muscles are incredibly important for injury prevention. According to the American Chiropractic Association, over half of Americans experience low back pain. And those 31 million people spend about $50 billion dollars a year in search of a cure! Good posture and strong core muscles can absolutely help you alleviate your pain, if it comes from a mechanical (not medical) issue.*

4. **Bodyweight exercises can be done anywhere!**

In the photos below, you will see me performing the exercises, outside, with a mat and park bench. Because these exercises don't require any equipment, besides your body, you can get your workout in at home or while travelling! No excuses! You can have a great, full-body workout, wherever you are!

5. **Bodyweight exercises lower your injury potential**

- **Additional weight can cause us to use momentum, rather than control.**

Many people, particularly on the release of an exercise, will allow momentum to take over to drop the weight, release the pulley, come down to the floor, etc. Without extreme control, momentum becomes the driving force. When that happens, correct form is lost and injury potential increases.

- **Additional weight can add pressure to bones and joints.**

Adding weight to an exercise adds pressure to the body. For some people, especially older women, women with arthritis, or women with osteoporosis, this is extremely uncomfortable, and even dangerous! Resistance training, however, has been shown to be an effective form of strength training to increase bone density. Bodyweight exercise are a great for this because they require no additional weight and are able to be controlled more easily.

- **Much of joint pain comes from misalignment, or an imbalance in the body.**

Strengthening muscles around the joint can help correct that misalignment. So, strength training is crucial. However, if we add additional weight to an already misaligned, weak area, the potential for injury increases. Body imbalances and misalignments also lead to less efficient movement, increasing injury potential not just in the target area, but throughout the body! Bodyweight exercises give us the opportunity to create stronger muscles, without risking the health of our joints.

Performing Bodyweight Exercises

Many barre and Pilates mat classes use light weights, seeking to increase your workout. Mine don't. In fact, when I created CA**BARRE**T, I made a very conscious decision NOT to use props.

Why? As you just read, there are plenty of issues to be aware of when you add weights into a moving exercise. And also, because you can actually get more of a workout when you perform bodyweight exercises! The catch, of course, is that you have to perform them correctly!

As I mentioned above, there are a few things that you need to do to check your bodyweight exercise form. I love lists and bullet-points. They give me a very concrete way to make sure I'm getting everything done!

So, I've created one for you as you go through your bodyweight exercises. And the best part-- only 3 steps! Totally easy to do and remember!

Your Bodyweight Exercise Checklist

1. **Engage your postural muscles.**
   Pull your navel to your spine and drop your tailbone towards your heels. Pull your shoulders down and back. Imagine a zipper between the two sides of your ribcage in the front, so your upper abdominals are engaged. If you have done all of this, you should feel tight, but lifted, in your core. Moving with control means controlling even the parts of the body that are NOT moving!

2. **Work with resistance, not momentum.**
   Remember, we are doing the movement AND resisting it, to make long, lean, strong and flexible muscles. To help with that--

3. **Use your imagination.**
   This engages your mind and your body. Focus on your movements, execute them with control, and you will have a more effective workout. Joseph Pilates, the creator of Pilates, used to say "It is the mind that guides the body." He knew keeping your mind focused would lead to a deeper workout!

69

This also increases your brain/body communication skills, which is important for motor control, injury prevention and rehabilitation. (See this study from Elon University on the importance of undistracted, focused exercise: http://www.elon.edu/e-net/Article/41203)

Over the next few pages, I'm going to give you instructions and images to help you create a bodyweight exercise regimen. See if you can identify the 3 steps from our Bodyweight Exercise Checklist in each one!

Together, we will look at arms, abs, glutes and thighs. But these are just examples. Remember, you can use the Bodyweight Exercise Checklist to on any bodyweight exercise. In fact, I encourage you to apply it to all of your traditional weight-loaded exercises. See if you notice a difference!

Arms- Bicep Curls

- Hold your arms out straight in front of your shoulders, palms up. Stand tall, stomach pulled in, shoulders down. **(Image 1a)**

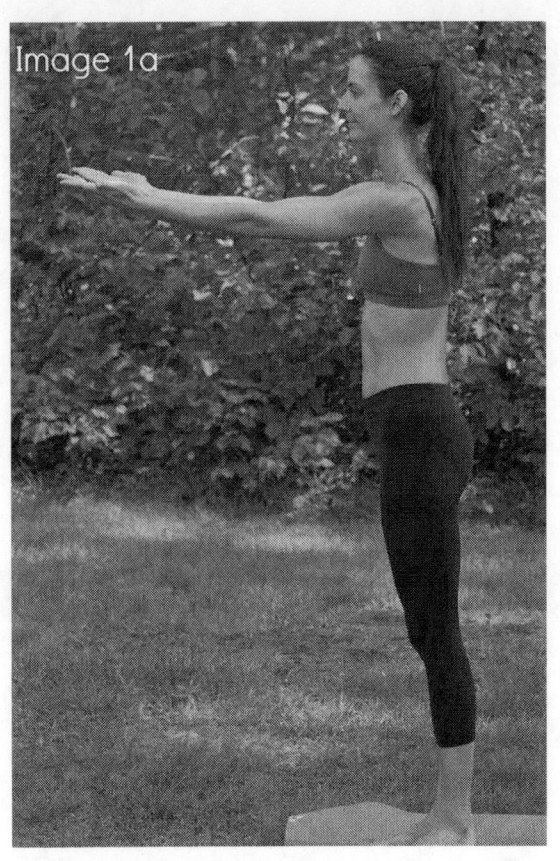

Image 1a

Imagine 100lb weights in your hands.

- Keeping your elbows in line with your shoulders, bend them, so your hands come towards you.

  Can you feel the weight? Feel your bicep strengthening here!

  Continue pulling your lower arms up, so your elbows are at 90 degrees, with your wrists in right over your elbows. **(Image 1b)**

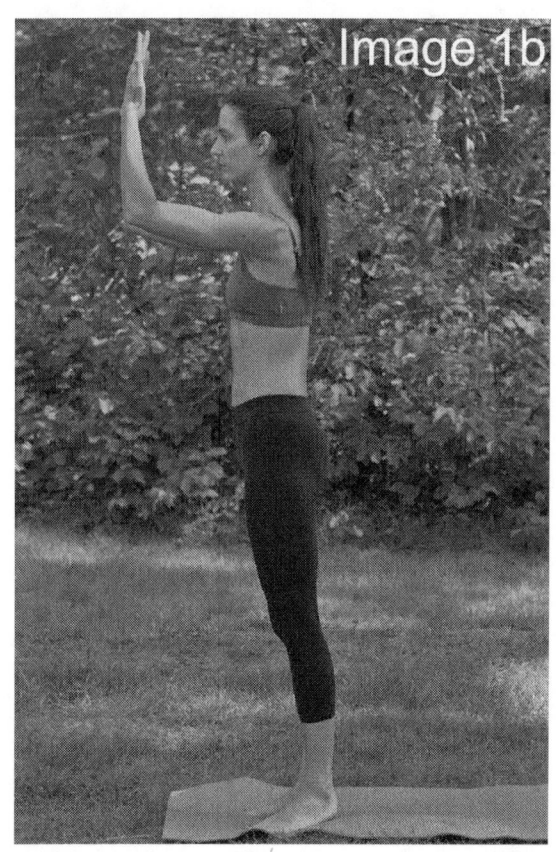

- Continuing to keep your elbows up, stomach in, shoulders down, press your hands back down to where you began.
  Feel the bicep lengthen, and your tricep strengthen.
- Repetitions- 3-5
- Alternate Image- *If the weight in the hands image isn't working for you, try this- your personal trainer, or a football player, or Arnold Schwarzenegger, is standing in front of you. He has his hands on top of yours. To pull in to 90 degrees, you must also pull his hands up. To press back down, imagine his hands on the back of yours. You must now push him away.*

Abs- Roll Down

- Sit on the floor with your legs together, knees bent, feet flat on the floor. Put your hands in the back of your knees.
Draw your navel into your spine, so your back is rounded.
(Image 2a)

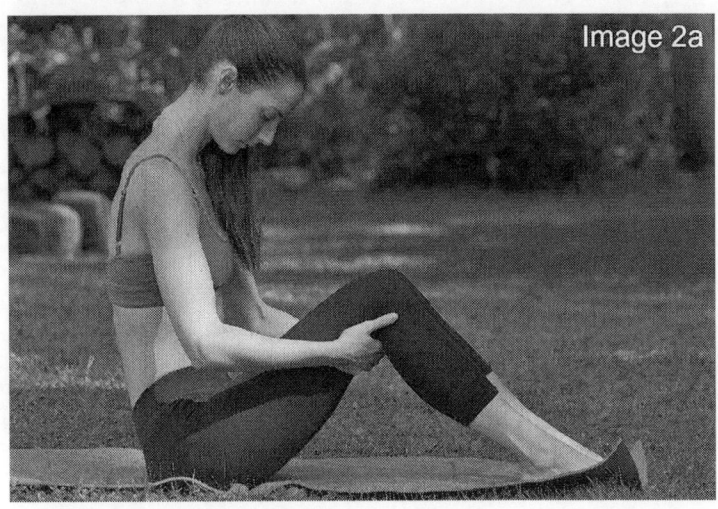

Not your shoulders! Your back.

- Pulling your abdominals in, begin to roll down to the floor. Roll back just until your arms are straight. **(Image 2b)**

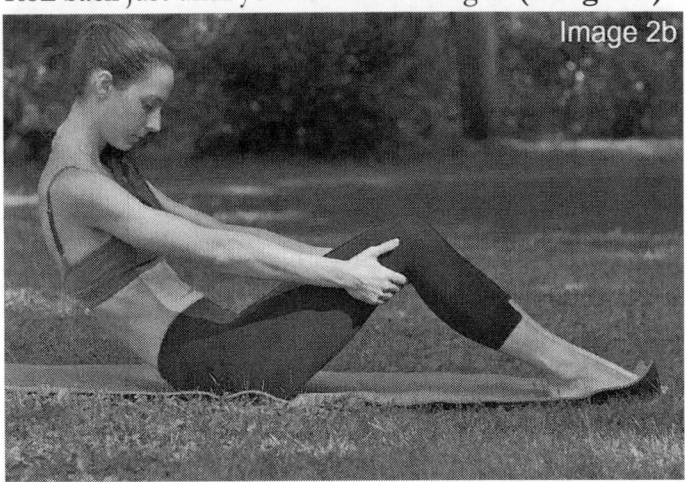

Imagine a string, pulling your navel through your spine and back into the floor.

- Hold it there for a 3-count. *Can you feel your abdominal muscles holding you in place?*
- Roll back up to you starting position, using your abdominals to lift, NOT using your arms to pull!
- Repetitions- 6-10
- Progress it- Roll down further (to your ribcage, or the tips of your shoulder blades, or even the whole way).
- NOTE- *Alway be sure it is your abdominal muscles moving you, whether you are going forward or back. You are not letting gravity push you down, or using momentum or your arms to come back up. Work only from the center.*

Thighs- Plies

- Plie is a ballet term that means- To bend.
- Set-up- Stand facing a ballet barre or chair. Only 2 fingers of each hand are on the barre/chair. It is there just to assist with balance, not to hold you up! **(Image 3a)**

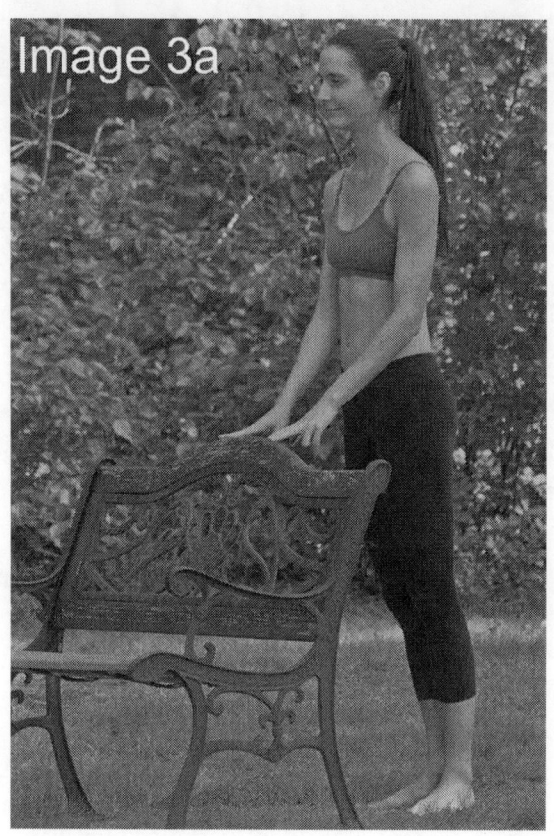

Image 3a

- Begin with your heels together and toes apart. This way, as you bend your knees, they will be in line with your feet, preventing torque on the knee.
- Draw your navel into your spine and lift your spine through the top of your head, standing as tall as you can.
- Begin to bend your knees, keeping your heels on the floor. Take a 4-count to go as low as you possibly can. **(Image 3b)**

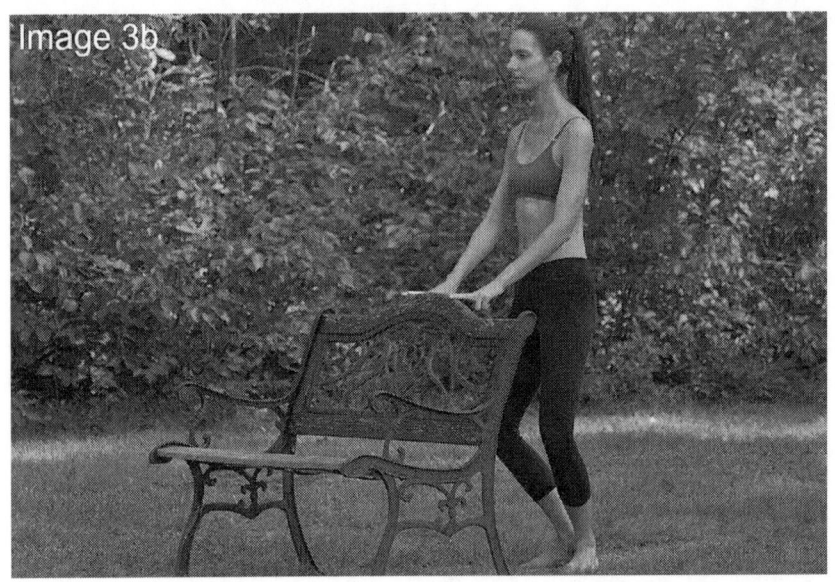

Image 3b

Imagine your bottom and stomach still lifting up as you go down to create the resistance. Imagine your knees being pulled out to the side, rather than just bending- feel how that works your thighs more.

- Make sure you are not sticking your seat out behind you (this will strain your low back) or dropping your upper body over (you will miss the good core work)!
- Come back to standing in a 4-count.
  Imagine your inner thighs being pulled together rather than just your knees unbending. Feel your stomach and your bottom lift even higher.
- Repetitions- 8 times
- Progress it- Do the exercise free standing. This increases your core work, as you have to balance. Plus, you'll get extra arm work if you hold your arms up and out to the side!

Thighs- Tendus

- Tendu is a ballet term that means- To stretch.
- Set-up- Stand facing a ballet barre or chair. Only 2 fingers of each hand are on the barre/chair. It is there just to assist with balance, not to hold you up! **(Image 4a)**

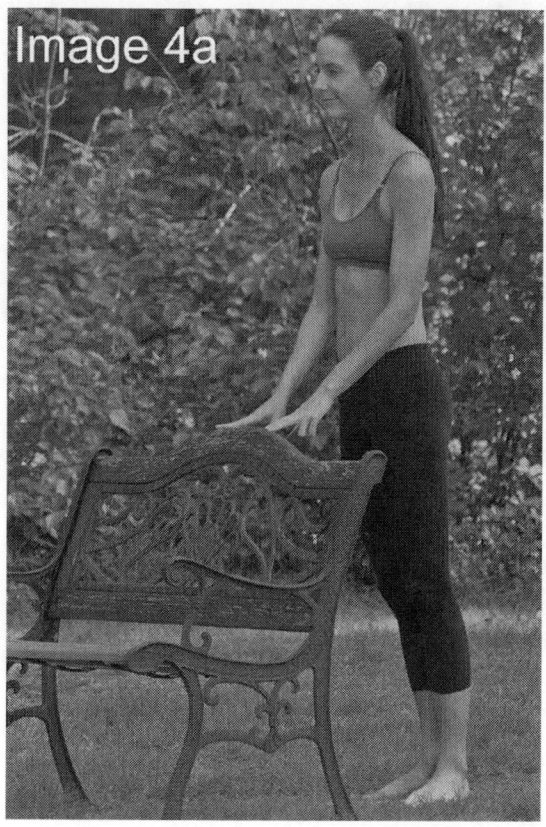

- Begin with your heels together and toes apart. This way, as you bend your knees, they will be in line with your feet, preventing torque on the knee.
- Draw your navel into your spine and lift your spine through the top of your head, standing as tall as you can.

- Begin to bend your knees, keeping your heels on the floor. Take a 4-count to go as low as you possibly can. **(Image 4b)**

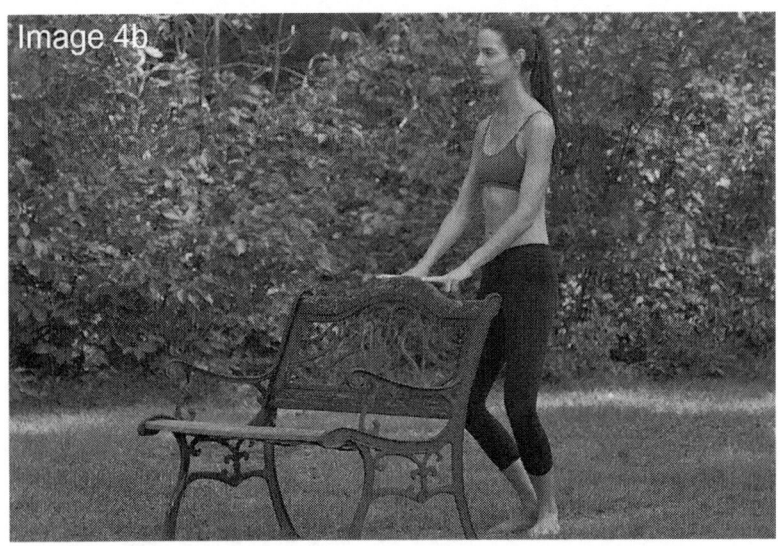

Image 4b

Imagine your bottom and stomach still lifting up as you go down to create the resistance. Imagine your knees being pulled out to the side, rather than just bending- feel how that works your thighs more.

- Make sure you are not sticking your seat out behind you (this will strain your low back) or dropping your upper body over (you will miss the good core work)!
- Stretch your right leg out to the side, while keeping your left leg in plie.

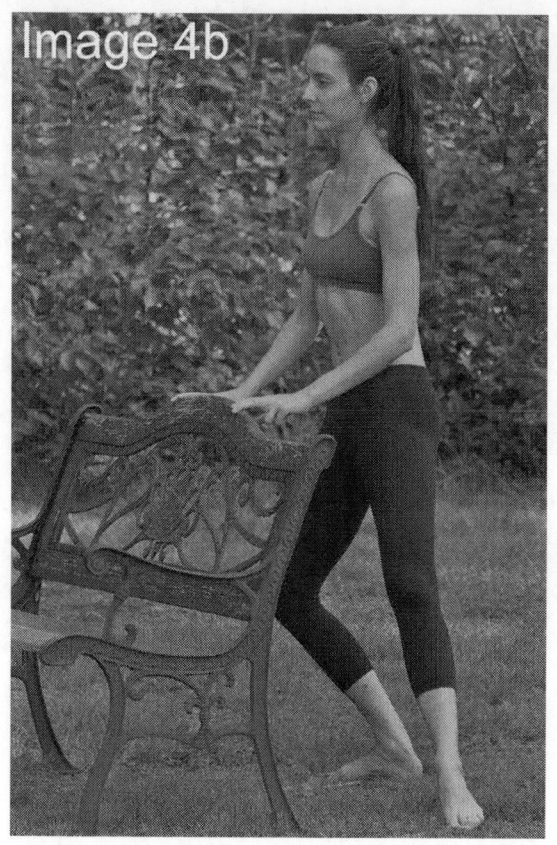

Image 4b

Imagine that rubber band around your ankles again. You have to press it open, stretching that right leg the whole way out!

- Draw your right leg back in, without standing up on the left. *Imagine pulling that rubber band closed. Don't let it snap. Drag that right foot in, and keep the left leg in plie.*
- Repetitions- 8 times on each leg.
- Progress it- Do the exercise free standing. This increases your core work, as you have to balance. Lift the arms up and out to the sides for bonus arm work! **(Image 4c)**

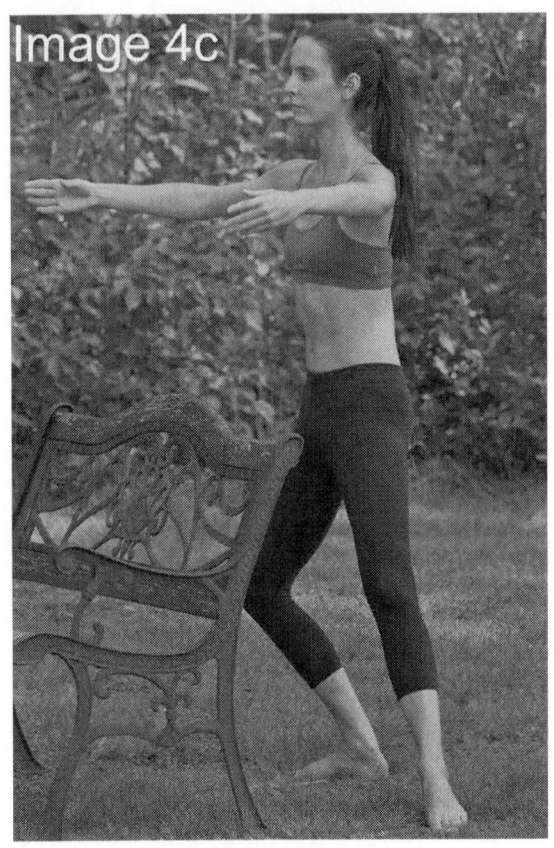

Glutes- Arabesque Leg Lift to the Back

- Arabesque is a ballet term that means- A pose on 1 leg, with a straight leg in the air.
- Set-up- Stand facing a ballet barre or chair. Only 2 fingers of each hand are on the barre/chair. It is there just to assist with balance, not to hold you up! **(Image 5a)**

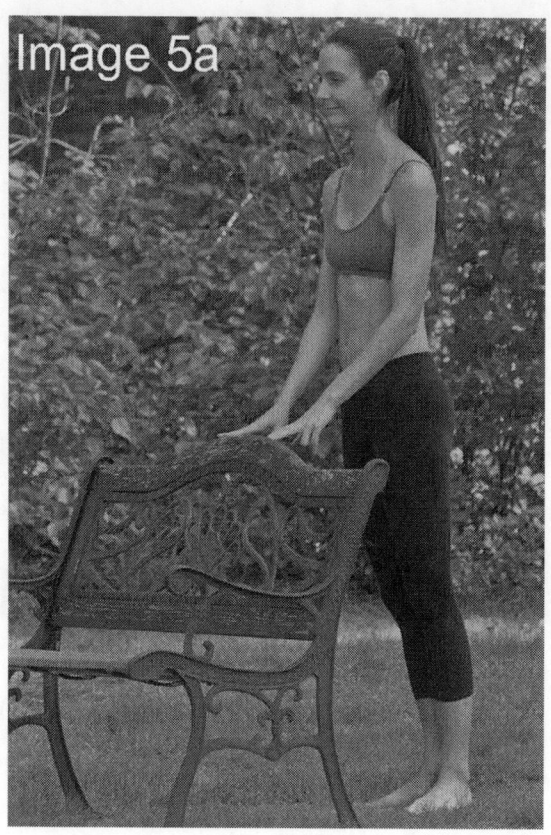

Image 5a

- Begin with your right leg extended behind you, with your toes on the floor.
- Draw your navel into your spine to support your back. This is very important to prevent low back strain in this exercise! You'll know you are doing this correctly if you keep your body upright, not dropped over towards the barre. If you feel a strain in your low back, engage and lift your abdominals more.
- Pull your right leg up behind you with control, taking a 4-count to reach your highest point. **(Image 5b)**

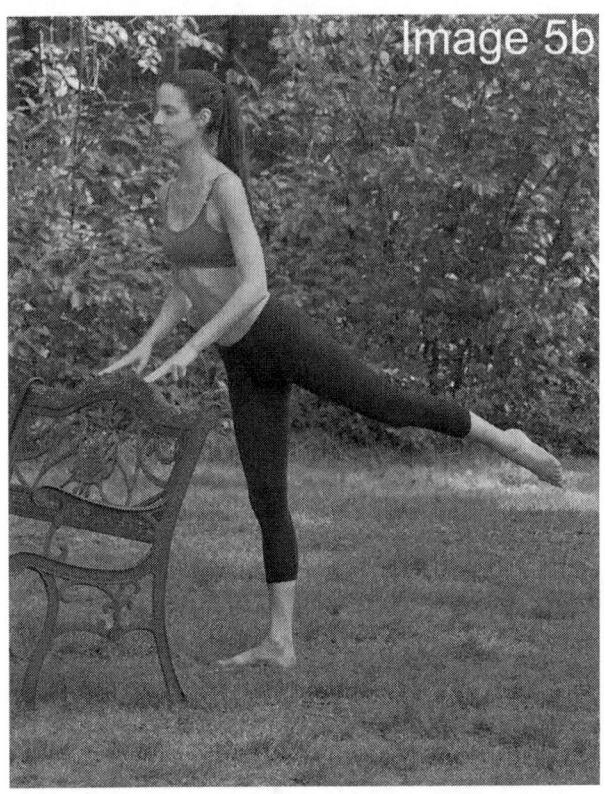

Imagine there is a big rubber band around your ankles, and you are pulling it apart as you lift your leg.

- Press the right leg back down to your starting position taking a 4-count to do so.

  Don't let the rubber band snap in. Slowly press it closed.

- Repetitions- 4 times on each leg.
- Progress it- Do the exercise free standing. This increases your core work, as you have to balance. Lift the arms up and out to the sides for bonus arm work! **(Image 5c)**

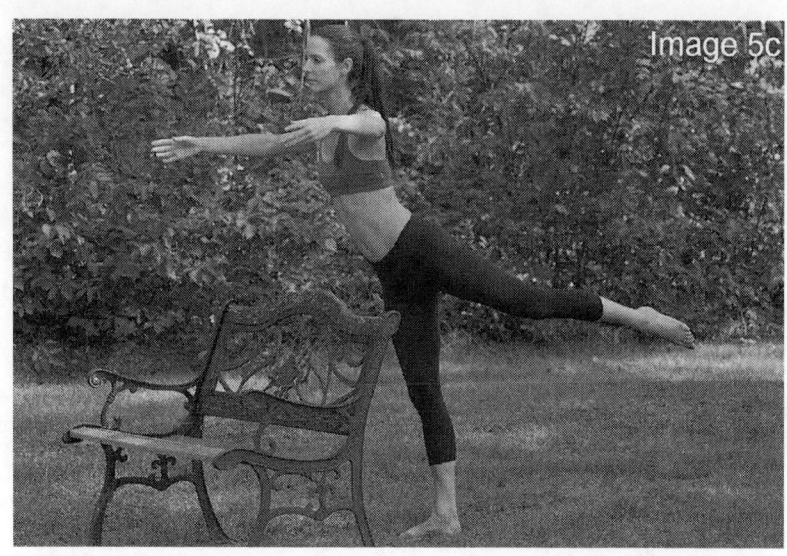

Bodyweight and Resistance Exercise- The Key word is INCREASE

We use resistance exercises as a form of strength training. As our muscles strengthen and tone, we are increasing our muscle mass. Increased muscle mass means an increased ability for the body to burn calories, even when not working out!

When we work with resistance, we engage our muscles in both contraction and extension, creating a double workout. We lengthen our muscles as we strengthen them, so we increase flexibility, as well as strength!

The above bodyweight exercises will definitely NOT bulk you up, but will build strength in long, lean muscles.

In these exercises, we are also working against gravity- either resisting it or pressing against it, and often both, at the same time, in different body parts!

In every exercise above, we are working to keep the core engaged and lifted, increasing our strength and benefiting our posture. The roll down, which is core specific, targets those postural muscles even more deeply.

All of the above bodyweight exercises will not only work the target body part, but will have you working from the center, out. This is a huge plus of bodyweight exercises- they are for your whole body!

One final benefit of bodyweight exercises- these will increase your mind/body connection.

Because we are really engaging our mind, to create images with our exercises, and to check in with our bodies, as we go through the movements, we are increasing the communication between our brain and our muscles.

This is especially important for learning to FEEL proper form in the body, discover the difference between discomfort and pain, and most significantly, to prevent injuries.

Clear pathways between the brain and muscles are helpful for rapid response in a dangerous situation-- stepping out of the way of a falling object or on-coming child on a skateboard, for example.

These clear pathways also make for better and more efficient execution of everyday activities, as you practice proper muscle recruitment, you decrease the chances for overuse injury .

I hope your knowledge and practice of bodyweight exercises has been furthered by this chapter. If you are looking for a few more exercise ideas, then you have FREE ACCESS to my CA**BARRE**T video - The Thigh Toning Booty Blasting Leg Series.:

http://cabarretfit.com/cabarret-10-minute-thigh-toning-booty-blasting

This quick video will give you a great series of exercises that will have you using your bodyweight and resistance to increase strength and flexibility, and tone up your backside!

About Nicole LaBonde

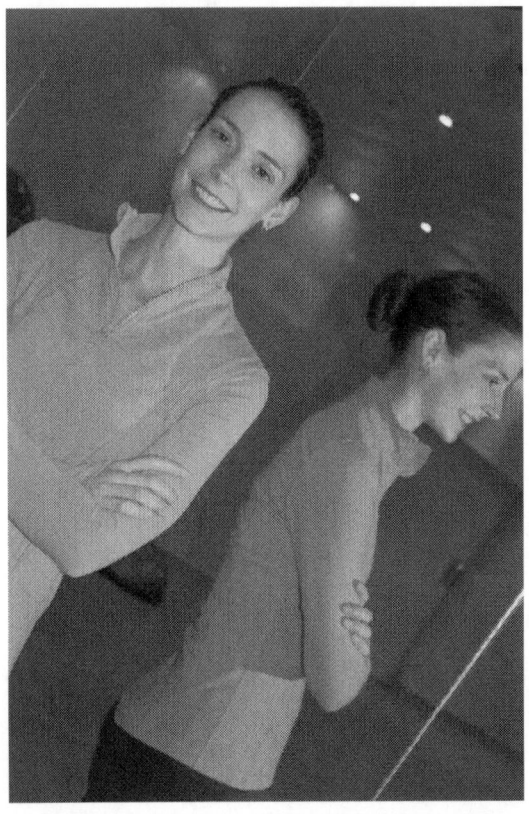

Nicole LaBonde is the Creatrix and Master Instructor of CA**BARRE**T a blend of strengthening barre work and cardio burlesque dance- a calorie-burning, muscle-sculpting, sexy workout! She teaches regularly in various locations in Miami, Florida.

Ms. LaBonde is also a certified instructor through the prestigious Romana's Pilates program. She teaches private and group Classical Pilates sessions at True Pilates Miami in Florida. Currently, she trains with Daria Pace, the daughter of Sari Mejia Santo and granddaughter of Romana Kryzanowska, proteges of Joseph Pilates himself.

Nicole fuels her body and her work with Isagenix products.

In addition to her fitness work, Nicole is a voice and presentation coach, at Public Persona, LLC, specializing in helping yoga teachers, fitness instructors, life coaches and healers protect their voices and create and deliver client-attracting presentations.

Learn more at nicolelabonde.com or cabarretfit.com or www.publicpersonallc.com or www.nicolelabonde.isagenix.com.
On Facebook www.facebook.com/cabarretfit
On Twitter @cabarretfit

All photos by Valerie D. Perry (www.valeriedperry.com)

CHAPTER 4

Danielle Vernon

Core Bodyweight Exercises for Women

Tone up anytime, anywhere by just using your own body weight

Introduction:

We watch what we eat. We try to sleep 8 hours a night. We attempt to drink 8-8 oz glasses of water per day and we focus our goals on staying as healthy as possible. This means, hopefully finding work-life balance and making room for an active lifestyle.

If you're reading this book, you are obviously one of these people that cares about their body but maybe doesn't quite know how to get started. Or, maybe, you've been down that road of gym memberships that don't get used and you're looking for something different.

Let's face it, doing the same exercises day in and day out gets boring for even the most motivated of us. Perhaps you're struggling to find time, between your family and work, to get out for that cardio workout or to go to the gym consistently. Perhaps you travel and aren't able to be as consistent as you'd like.

Now there's an easier way to stay on track with your work-out routine and shake things up at the same time. You don't need an expensive gym membership to sculpt a great body.

As a woman, I understand that most of us are concerned about developing too muscular a physique. The reality is that the average woman simply does not usually produce the testosterone necessary to build big, bulky muscles. Exercise using your body weight will naturally will give you the sleek, healthy body and improved posture you're looking for that will make you not only feel better and more confident but look taller and slimmer as well.

Using your own body weight is not only convenient and efficient but it requires very little extra equipment. Keep your core strong, your body toned and strong by using what god gave you....your own body. As you progress, you can then start to add in extra challenges using tools like hand and ankle weights, therapy balls and a BOSU.

With almost 15 years of experience in treating patients and athletes of all ages, suffering from deconditioning, muscle and joint problems, the most successful, and long-lasting, outcomes result when an exercise program includes both active strength movements as well as simultaneous stabilization components.

For women, it is especially important to include both strength-training components (to improve fat burning) and stabilization components to maximize muscle activation around the joints so that we can tone those trouble zones. (you know what I'm talking about ladies....the dreaded muffin top, wiggly under-arms, thigh flab and "old lady hump" known also as Dowager's hump).

This program combines a variety of movements into one workout that maximizes muscle use throughout our body with only a few positions. It will tone your core while, simultaneously, improving your posture and strength of our arms (stabilizing from the shoulder) and legs (stabilizing from the hips).

With these 8 simple body weight exercises that take less than 20 minutes, you can tone your arms, legs, core, improve your posture and burn fat anywhere, anytime.

When you consider the added benefit of being able to do it anytime, anywhere and in a short period of time, the only question is.....what's stopping you?

Why are core exercises so important?

Let's start by looking at your spine

A healthy back has three natural curves:

- An inward or forward curve at the neck (cervical curve)
- An outward or backward curve at the upper back (thoracic curve)
- An inward curve at the lower back (lumbar curve)

Good core strength leads to a strong posture which helps to maintain these natural curves, while a weak abdomen will worsen poor posture which can lead to too much tightness along the front of our bodies and too much length and weakness along the back of our bodies.

This leads to excessive and unnecessary stresses or pulling on muscles which lead to pain. In addition, our seating throughout the day (at home, at our office, in our car, at the movies, in a meeting....you name it) is usually poorly fitting and forces us into staying in this slumped position.

How do you rate on the wall test?

To test your standing posture, take the wall test. Stand with your head, shoulder blades and buttocks touching a wall, and have your heels about 2 to 4 inches (about 5 to 10 centimeters) away from the wall. Place your arms on the wall with your elbows bent and rotate your arms away from your body until the back of your hands touch the wall.

Now, try to keep your elbows and back of hands on the wall as you bring your arms up overhead (as if you were doing a snow angel).

If you have overly tight chest muscles and weak postural balance, you will not be able to keep the back of your hands and your elbows on the wall while still maintaining a good contact between the wall and your low back/buttocks.

Why does this matter?
Research is growing that many of our health conditions may stem from deficiencies in our posture (excessive pressure on our diaphragm, neck, head, shoulders and back not to mention our lungs, heart and organs). Poor posture has even been shown to contribute to increased mortality rates, poor self-esteem, and decreased work efficiency.

The Journal of the American the American Medical Association has found that people who sit the most and perform no weekly physical activity having the highest all-cause mortality risk.

Weight training can also be beneficial for women because resistance exercises help increase bone density, which may in turn help prevent or slow the development of osteoporosis.

Lastly, it is important to note that these exercises will be critically helpful in allowing us to improve and maintain a healthy posture which can effect everything else that we do, day in and day out.

NOTE: *Please remember, if you have any medical conditions that you think may be irritated or exacerbated by starting a new program, you should always make sure you are cleared by your doctor to participate.*

How do I know where to start?
Beginning a new or different program, if you've never exercised consistently before, can be an overwhelming task. Knowing how to set goals can be even more confusing without the proper direction.

As a physical therapist, I see people come in to my clinic all the time that have overdone it because they've listened to their neighbor, their friends or a stranger tell them what they should do and how they should do it. The reality is that we are all different. You can't take someone else's experience and expect that your body will react the same way as theirs.

With this in mind, if you are doing the exercises correctly, you should expect to feel some muscle soreness within 1-2 days afterwards. This is called DOMS or delayed onset muscle soreness. If you don't feel this soreness, you are likely not challenging your muscles enough so that they will recover in a stronger, more efficient structure the next time you need them.

It is important that you find that fine line between 1-2 day delayed onset muscle soreness and working too aggressively that creates trauma to the muscle for more than 1-2 days. If soreness persists beyond 1-2 days, or you notice any unusual swelling, contact your doctor.

As you get fitter with body-weight training, you will be able to perform more repetitions of a given exercise, but since the weight you are working with remains constant, your muscles will become conditioned and more defined as opposed to larger.

Basic Terms:

Muscle tone
Muscle tone is essentially how much tension (or readiness to react) a particular muscle holds, so it's important to build up the muscle groups you are aiming to tone.
Building lean muscle mass is often overlooked in the quest for tone, but along with losing an appropriate amount of fat, it's really the only way to see any significant progress. The most effective method is to combine different kinds of workouts in order to build up your lean muscle and cut down extra fat.

You need to plan on giving this program 6-8 to truly see the effect that your exercise will have on your body. Research supports that it takes 8-10,000 repetitions to re-educate a muscle so get out your calendar, a chart, a note pad, your phone app etc and lots of patience. Start on

Day 1 by tracking what you do and how much you're doing. It will help you to see your progress when your motivation starts to wane.

Repetitions
Repetitions refer to the number of times you perform an exercise in sequence without stopping. For example, repeat a movement x10.

Sets
Sets refer to the amount of times you perform these groups of repetitions, usually with a 1-2 minute break in between for recovery. For example, performing 10 repetitions with a rest break will be considered one set. You will perform 10 repetitions a second time, rest and perform 10 more repetitions and rest. This would be considered 3 sets of 10 repetitions.

Intensity
For our purposes here, the term "intensity" is what fatigues the muscles and creates change and growth so that it can adapt to the same stress more efficiently the next time it is taxed. This is what will ultimately change your body, what's going to help develop that muscle mass. Increasing your metabolism will then come once you've got your distance set and you increase your intensity so as to challenge your body to perform at a higher level.

Getting started:

When you perform the 8 exercises below, keep in mind that you are trying to complete 3 sets of 10 repetitions but, if starting at the correct resistance, you might only be able to perform 10 on the first set, 7 on the second set and 5 on the third set before you fatigue the muscles.

This is perfectly normal and indicates that you are working at the correct level to maximally challenge your muscle. If you are able to complete 3 sets of 10 without muscle fatigue, the activity is probably too easy for you and your muscle will not have to adapt and change to become stronger.

As you can achieve 3 sets of 10, increase your goal to 3 sets of 15 then 3 sets of 20. Once you are able to complete 3 sets of 20 with good

94

form and minimal fatigue, it's time to return to 3 sets of 10 and add a 4th set, working your way up to five sets of 10, 15 then 20.

The first step to your program will be to use these numbers as a guideline towards which you want to achieve but the most important thing is to fatigue the muscle.

The exercises in this program attempt to include areas that work every major muscle group: legs, including quadriceps, hamstrings and calves; chest; back; shoulders; arms; and the core, which includes the abdominals, lower back and gluts.

The core is especially important because it is the "powerhouse" of the body. The shoulder blades are especially important because they are the "anchor" of our arms. Both these areas provide stability, leverage and strength for any physical activity we carry out during our normal, functioning day.

What if you're already in good shape?

Women that are already lean but need to improve their muscular definition will also find this routine a good option. Incorporate this total-body workout into your schedule at least twice a week for 20 minutes.

This program is made up of "compound" movements which require you to multi-task so that you are getting both arm and leg movements engaged simultaneously.

These exercises not only help you build muscle and tone, but rev-up your metabolism by working several muscle groups simultaneously. In the beginning you can perform these exercises with nothing but yourself and a mat.

As you start to progress your routine, adding a set of dumbbells, medicine ball, stability ball and BOSU ball will continue to give you limitless options to challenge yourself and tone all areas of your body.

Warm Up

Preparing your muscles by warming up before a workout improves performance and reduces the risk of injury. A study published in the August 2006 issue of the "Journal of Strength & Conditioning Research" suggests that a dynamic warm-up is more effective in improving power and agility than just stretching. Get your body ready for the main workout with around 10 minutes of activities such as skipping, stair jumps or jogging on the spot before performing stretching movements for each body part.

Cardiovascular exercise has shown to be particularly important for an overall female fitness because it helps burn fat and creates a leaner silhouette as well as strengthening the heart and lungs. But we also know that lifting weight creates a fat burn in our muscles that can last up to 4-5 hours after we've finished working.

Biking, fitness walking, skipping and elliptical are all good options for cardiovascular exercise. Swimming is a terrific overall body conditioning exercise. Running, in particular, 30 second sprints followed by a 10 second rest, done in sets of 8 (3-4x/week) have been shown to build lean muscle mass in the legs, buttocks and abs.

According to a 2009 study in the Journal of Strength and Conditioning Research, they also kickstart a fat-burning hormonal reaction. These two factors combine to make sprints a secret weapon in getting toned up quickly.

Performing cardio workouts at least 3-4 times a week for 30 minutes (unless you're performing sprints) will keep your metabolism revved up and burning fat.

Don't forget about your nutrition:

Our bodies need good food, plenty of water and protein in order for the muscles to maximally recover and re-build stronger. Eat a nutritious, low-fat diet that minimizes fast food, processed foods and foods that are high in saturated and trans fats. Incorporate a variety of fresh fruits, vegetables, whole grains, lean meats and low-fat dairy products into your diet to improve your overall health, lose fat and build lean muscle.

If you are vegan or vegetarian, substitute lentils, soy, beans and nuts for protein and calcium sources. Don't forget that eating 5-6 smaller meals a day will keep our insulin levels from spiking (when we eat a lot) and dipping (when we go too long without eating) which cause our insulin to store fat as a protective measure.

Make healthy lifestyle choices by avoiding or quitting smoking, drinking and other high-risk habits. Get at least eight hours of sleep a night and take time to relax every day.

Let's get started

1. Squats with bicep curl

   Stand with your feet spread shoulder-width apart. Place your weights at your side and, as you squat, bring the weights up towards your shoulders. Slightly rotate so that your pinkie finger is moving towards your shoulder. This slight rotation will incorporate all 3 muscles that make up your forearm flexors. Bend your knees so that you are pushing your hips back but don't allow your knees to go beyond your toes. Pause, then slowly push yourself back to a standing position.

   Progressions:

   i.   Have one foot up on a surface behind you. Perform your 10 repetitions and switch to the other leg.
   ii. Place one foot on an uneven surface such as a BOSU.
   iii. Stand with both feet on an unstable surface ie. foam pad or flat side of a BOSU.

2. Chair dips target your triceps but is a good source of stabilization for your upper extremity and core as well.

Start by placing your hands, palms facing behind you, on a flat surface, such as a chair, with your body positioned straight in front of the chair. Place your feet either on the ground, with your knees bent. Lower your body by bending your elbows, keeping your feet stationary, and descending until your upper arms reach parallel to the ground. Do not let your shoulders dip lower than your hands. Reverse the movement by pressing your body upward until you return to your starting position.

Progressions:

i. Straighten your legs out in front of you. Keep your hips up as you bend your arms.
ii. Place feet on another raised surface a few feet away.
iii. Place feet on an unstable surface such as a ball or BOSU.

3. Lunge with military press

Stand with your feet hip-width apart and your weights by your side. **With your legs:** Step forward with your right leg and slowly lower your body until your right knee is bent at least 90 degrees but doesn't go beyond the end of your toes. Pause, then raise up and bring your back foot forward so that you move forward (like you're walking) a step with every rep. Alternate the leg you step forward with each time. **With your arms:** As you step into a lunge with your legs you will press the weight up overhead and meet the weights above your head. As you stand to take the next step forward, you will slowly lower the weights back to your side.

Progressions:

i. Have one foot up on an unstable surface such as the BOSU.

ii. Raise only one arm (opposite to the leg that is forward) at a time. This will work more of your oblique muscles

iii. Step up on a step to finish your lunge. Press the weight overhead as you step up.

4. ¼ squats with diagonal shoulder press

Stand with both legs shoulder width apart. With a weight in both hands, reach down towards your right foot as you perform a ¼ squat and, as your return, bring the weight up and over your left shoulder as if you were going to throw it. This will create a complete diagonal movement. Perform your repetitions on this side and then change the diagonal direction.

Progressions:

i. Stand on one leg with shoes on and use the opposite hand to diagonally shift the weight.

ii. Perform single leg version without shoes on.

iii. Perform exercise standing on both legs on an unstable surface such as a BOSU.

5. Plank with alternate leg lift

Assume a pushup position off your elbows and your knees so that you are creating as straight a surface between your shoulders and your knees as possible. Lift one leg off the floor and slowly extend that leg back behind you as if you were trying to reach the back wall. Return it underneath you being aware of not twisting at your hips and lift the other leg. That's one rep.

Progressions:

i. Straighten your legs and balance between your toes and your forearms

ii. Straighten your arms and balance between your toes and your hands

Perform this activity with your arms supported on either side of a BOSU

6. Plank with diagonal crunch

Assume a pushup position with your arms straight and your feet, shoulder width, on the floor. Try to create as flat a surface along your body as possible. Lift one leg off the floor and slowly bring the knee towards your opposite shoulder. Return it to the starting position and do the same thing with your opposite leg. That's one rep.

Progressions:

i.   Bring your feet together so they are touching thereby reducing your base of support.
ii. Perform this activity with your hands supported on either side of a BOSU.
iii. Keep your arms straight and core engaged, shift your weight onto your left arm, rotate your torso to the right, and raise your right arm toward the ceiling so that your body forms a T; your right foot should now be on top of your left. Pause for three seconds, then return to the starting position and repeat on the other side. That's one rep.

7. Side plank with leg lift

Assume a pushup position off your elbows and your knees then turn onto one side so that only one knee and its same side elbow are supporting you. Keep your hips up so that you are creating as straight a surface between your shoulders and your knees as possible. Lift your top leg, straighten it then lift it up towards the ceiling. Keep it in line with your bottom leg. Do not let if drift forward of your bottom leg or you will be using more of your hip flexors than your side gluts. Keep your hips from rotating as you slowly return leg back to your side.

Perform all your reps on one side and then turn onto the opposite side.

Progressions:

  i. Straighten your legs and balance between your toes and your forearms as you lift the upper leg.
 ii. Straighten your arms and balance between your toes and your hands while you maintain a strong, stable core and lift your leg up towards the ceiling.
iii. Perform this activity off your feet with your arm straight. Lift your leg up, bring it back down to neutral (without resting it on your lower leg), move it forward of your body about 60 degrees, return it back to neutral and then leg it down on your lower leg. This is one rep.

8. Close hand Push-ups

Leaning against a wall, place your feet about 12 inches from the wall and your hands shoulder height and 4 inches apart (this works your triceps harder). Keep your body straight (don't let your hips sag) as you lower yourself towards the wall. Keep your head up and lower yourself until your chest nearly touches the wall. Count to 3 as your lower yourself towards the wall and count to 5 as you bring yourself back from the wall (this will work all your stabilization muscles around the shoulder blade to their fullest if you move more slowly on the return). Keep your elbows tucked close to your sides as you lower your body.

Progressions:

i. Place your feet further back to create a greater angle.
ii. Add a ball under your hands to provide an unstable base.

iii.   Find a lower surface like a counter top or chair and progress towards being able to do it on the floor. In addition, as you start to lower the surface from which you're doing a push-up, start on your knees and only progress up on your toes when you can perform full repetitions.

It all adds up

All of the exercises in this program will be the most beneficial if they are paralleled with healthy lifestyle changes. If we take our time and effort to bring our bodies into a stronger, more toned alignment then we get into our cars and slouch, sit at our desks or on our sofas and slump, sleep in a fetal position, stand with bad posture, lean over our tables, counters, grocery carts.....fill in the blank.....then we are wasting our time. Our muscles are so confused that they will naturally revert back to our more normal, habitual weak state.

Tips for healthy lifestyle changes

1. **Drink lots of water.** We should try to get at least 8-8 oz glasses of water per day. This does not include the extra water we need while we're working out.
2. **Eat small meals.** 5-6 smaller meals a day is the best to keep up your energy and support the nutritional needs of your muscles as they recover, rather than 3 large meals a day.
3. **Stretch** your anterior hip (hip flexor stretch) and chest muscles (pec stretch) frequently throughout the day. NOTE: The effects of a stretch only last 1-2 hours so, if you're going to make consistent gains on a tight muscle, you can't just rely on stretching 1-2x/day to see program.
4. **Be consistent.** Support your posture at home, at work and in the car. If you are consistent, you'll start to see improvements in your body shape, tone and posture immediately and long-lasting benefits within 6-8 weeks.
5. **Give yourself a day in between to rest.** Your muscles need some time to recover and build new cross-bridges so that they

can produce more muscle contraction the next time force is required. So, if you're focusing on lower body exercises, work on upper body exercises the next day.

6. **Get up**....and out of your chair every hour and stretch your arms overhead and gently bounce backwards to improve the blood flow to your low back (lumbar extension stretch).

7. **Bring your environment closer** so that the surface that you're working with (keyboard or steering wheel) is as close as possible (and allowing for safety in the car) and your arms can hang relaxed by your side. This takes a significant amount of pressure off you're your neck and shoulders and will help to maintain the position you work so hard to obtain with your exercises.

8. **Adjust your standing work surfaces** so that you are not working over-top of your area but with your arms at 80-90 degrees of bend.

9. **Support your entire back, not just the lumbar area.** When you sit with an additional mid-back support, research shows that you can reduce the stress on your spine by up to 35%.

10. **Adjust your car seat.** We spend more and more time in our cars and have to consider how this static time decreases blood flow and postural awareness. For an optimal position, line your hips up with your knees. This will allow you to maintain your lumbar curve. Adding a mid-back support between your shoulder blades will bring you out of the contours of the seat and allow you to roll your shoulder blades back.

What's the big deal about posture?

You probably don't think much about posture, and if you do, you may believe it's just an aesthetics thing. Good posture looks better. It's a way to project a good impression.

Although this is true, good posture is far more than that. In fact, it's access to a lot of great stuff

1. Good posture gives you more energy.

When you have good posture, you can breathe deeper. Breathing deeper oxygenates the cells and gives you more physical energy.

Also, poor posture can restrict blood flow to your heart, lungs, and internal organs. This restricted flow negatively impacts your energy levels.

2. Good posture can help you breathe easier.

When you're hunched over, you physically restrict the ability of your diaphragm to expand which pushes air into your lungs. Your breath is your life force, so when you pinch it off, you not only decrease oxygen to your lungs but this, in turn, decreases nutrition to your organs and muscles.

3. Good posture makes you smarter.

When you can't get enough oxygen into your lungs, this will decrease the amount of oxygen available for your brain. Since your brain requires oxygen to work efficiently, good oxygen will make you feel attentive, alert and make fewer mistakes.

4. Good posture gives you more confidence.

It is difficult to impact your physical state without also impacting your mental state. If you look slumped, you're going to feel slumped. When you improve your posture, your sense of personal power will improve. Your self-esteem will improve and thus your outward appearance will be taller and stronger which will make you appear more confident to the people around you.

5. Good posture helps you get rid of excess weight.

Yep, it's true. Not only does good posture tend to make you look thinner, it can actually help you *be* thinner.

Believe it or not, slouching helps your body store fat. It does this because when you slouch, you impair your digestion and your glandular function. This happens because poor posture drops the rib cage onto your stomach, your intestines, and the organs located in your abdominal cavity.

Good posture is an easy and very important way to maintain a healthy mind and body. When you practice correct posture, your body is in alignment with your head over your shoulders.

This can alleviate common problems such as back or neck pain, headaches, and fatigue.

In conclusion:

Performing exercises that strengthen the muscles across your upper back and core will help you to maintain good posture and an overall healthier life. You don't need to develop a body builder physique to be healthy. Instead, this is more about building "muscle memory" so that you unconsciously and naturally maintain your correct posture without fatigue.

I have been a physical therapist for almost 15 years and with all my patients and athletes, regardless of physical ability, a strong core has always given them the best results. This is what led me to invent a back cushion that supported not only the low back but the entire spine in the same direction as our back muscles. This has allowed my patients to maintain the results they gain in physical therapy as they transition into their own day to day activity.

Please remember that these exercises are a general guideline based on the current research and my experience as an orthopedic sport and spine specialist. One program will not always suit everyone's needs. Please remember, if you have any medical conditions that you think may be irritated or exacerbated by starting this program, you should always make sure you are cleared by your doctor to participate.

Take your time, work within your abilities and have fun as you start to feel better in every part of your life. Good luck!

References:

1. 2008 Physical Activity Guidelines for Americans. U.S. Department of Health and Human Services. http://www.health.gov/paguidelines/guidelines/default.aspx. Accessed Feb. 1, 2013.
2. Kirk EP, et al. Minimal resistance training improves daily energy expenditure and fat oxidation. Medicine and Science in Sports and Exercise. 2009;41:1122.
3. Wilmore JH, et al. Physiology of Sport and Exercise. 4th ed. Champaign, Ill.: Human Kinetics; 2008:186.
4. Pollock ML, et al. Resistance training for health. The President's Council on Physical Fitness and Sports. https://www.presidentschallenge.org/informed/digest/docs/1996 12digest.pdf. Accessed Feb. 4, 2013.
5. Liu-Ambrose T, et al. Resistance training and executive functions: A 12-month randomized controlled trial. Archives of Internal Medicine. 2010;170:170.
6. "Journal of Strength & Conditioning Research"; Dynamic Vs.Static-Stretching Warm Up: the Effect on Power and Agility Performance; D.J. McMillan, et al.; Aug. 2006 - http://journals.lww.com/nsca-jscr/Abstract/2006/08000/Dynamic_Vs_Static_Stretching_Warm_Up__the_Effect.6.aspx
7. Frontera WR, et al. Essentials of Physical Medicine and Rehabilitation: Musculoskeletal Disorders, Pain, and Rehabilitation. 2nd ed. Philadelphia, Pa.: Saunders Elsevier; 2008. http://www.mdconsult.com/das/book/body/208746819-6/0/1678/0.html. Accessed April 10, 2012.
8. Kyphosis (roundback) of the spine. American Academy of Orthopaedic Surgeons. http://orthoinfo.aaos.org/topic.cfm?topic=A00423. Accessed April 10, 2012.
9. How to sit at a computer. American Academy of Orthopaedic Surgeons. http://orthoinfo.aaos.org/topic.cfm?topic=A00261. Accessed March 8, 2013.
10. Armiger P, et al. Stretching for Functional Flexibility. Philadelphia, Pa.: Lippincott Williams & Wilkins; 2010:171.
11. Tips to maintain good posture. American Chiropractic Association. http://www.acatoday.org/content_css.cfm?CID=1452. Accessed March 8, 2013.

12. Low back pain fact sheet. National Institute of Neurological Disorders and Stroke. http://www.ninds.nih.gov/health_and_medical/pubs/back_pain.htm. Accessed March 8, 2013.

13. Laskowski ER (expert opinion). Mayo Clinic, Rochester, Minn. March 11, 2013.

14. Sitting Time and All-Cause Mortality Risk in 222 497 Australian Adults, Hidde P. van der Ploeg, PhD; Tien Chey, MAppStats; Rosemary J. Korda, PhD; Emily Banks, MBBS, PhD; Adrian Bauman, MBBS, PhD *Arch Intern Med.* 2012;172(6):494-500. doi:10.1001/archinternmed.2011.2174

15. World Health Organization. *Global Health Risks: Mortality and Burden of Disease Attributable to Selected Major Risks.* Geneva, Switzerland: WHO Press; 2009

16. Brown WJ, Bauman AE, Owen N. Stand up, sit down, keep moving: turning circles in physical activity research? *Br J Sports Med.* 2009;43(2):86-88

17. Owen N, Bauman A, Brown W. Too much sitting: a novel and important predictor of chronic disease risk? *Br J Sports Med.* 2009;43(2):81-83

18. Tremblay MS, Colley RC, Saunders TJ, Healy GN, Owen N. Physiological and health implications of a sedentary lifestyle. *Appl Physiol Nutr Metab.* 2010;35(6):725-740

19. Van Uffelen JGZ, Wong J, Chau JY, et al. Occupational sitting and health risks: a systematic review. *Am J Prev Med.* 2010;39(4):379-388

Applied Ergonomics, Volume 38, Issue 6, November 2007, Pages 755–764. Effects of backrest design on biomechanics and comfort during seated work, Steven M. Carcone, Peter J. Keir., School of Kinesiology and Health Science, York University, Toronto, ON, Canada.

About Danielle Vernon

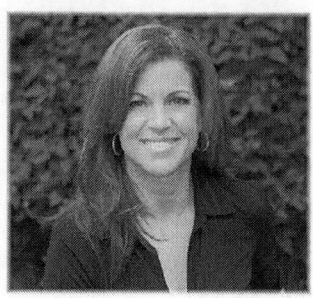 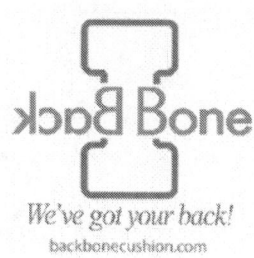

We've got your back!

backbonecushion.com

Danielle Vernon is a licensed orthopedic physical therapist with over 13 years of experience in treating sport and spine conditions. She is also the CEO of WorkWise Ergonomics Consulting, LLC and inventor of the Backbone Cushion™.

She is on the forefront of postural innovation and created the specialized back support device after a career orthopedic and industrial rehabilitation. She has worked with high level athletes and busy professionals, alike, to assist them to getting their bodies to their next desired level of health and function.

Ms. Vernon's leadership experience includes running multiple out-patient physical therapy and health facilities, developing and implementing on-site physical therapy and injury reduction program for 2,000+ Transit workers resulting in a $865,000 reduction in WC claims.

As a physical therapist, Ms. Vernon is experienced in treating a wide variety of patients ages 15-95, working with national sports teams in Canada and Chile and a stint with the LPGA.

She is a skilled therapist in hands-on methods related to orthopedic strain/sprain conditions, motor-vehicle accidents, total joint replacement, functional re-training, vestibular rehab, work conditioning, exercise strength and conditioning programs.

She has created and taught workshops on "The Prevention of Running Injuries," "Reducing Low-back Pain in High Mileage Drivers," "Assessment and Treatment of the Shoulder," "Managing Arthritis," and "Living with Osteoporosis." She is currently working on a book highlighting the importance of postural strength and core positioning titled "What you see is what you get: What does your posture say about you?"

She holds a BS in Physical Therapy from the University of Alberta and a BA in Psychology from the University of Ottawa and has completed over 20 specialized certifications in exercise rehabilitation, orthopedic physical assessment, ergonomics assessment and environmental ergonomics design.

She lives in beautiful Austin, Texas, and shares her free time between outdoor activities, friends, her church and volunteer work at Austin Pets Alive medical clinic and Dress for Success women's organization to help under-privileged women enter the work force.

CHAPTER 5

Buck Nimz

Important Bodyweight Exercises for Women

Why would a man be writing about bodyweight exercises for women? Because as a personal trainer, the majority of my clients have been women. And I will say this right up front: the ladies I've trained (and see training in the gym) out work most men. You ladies can teach men a thing or two about intensity, discipline and dedication when it comes to exercise.

Without a doubt one of the comments I get most often from women is: "I don't want to get big muscles." Men and women have the same types of muscles, but what makes a woman's muscle different from a man's is the metabolic hormonal actions that take place. Men have dominant levels of testerone, a powerful muscle building and fat burning hormone.

Women also have testerone but their levels of "T" are much lower than men. The woman's dominant hormone is estrogen, but even so, women still have some levels of testosterone.

Even if you have more than average, you're not going to get big man-like muscles but you can develop strong and powerful muscles and, pound-for-pound, you can even be stronger than a man. It's all about gender and genetics.

111

But what look do you like? Do you want to look like bodybuilder Cindy Johnson, or gymnast Shannon Miller, or marathon runner Catherine Ndereba, or fitness model Chassidy Luke?

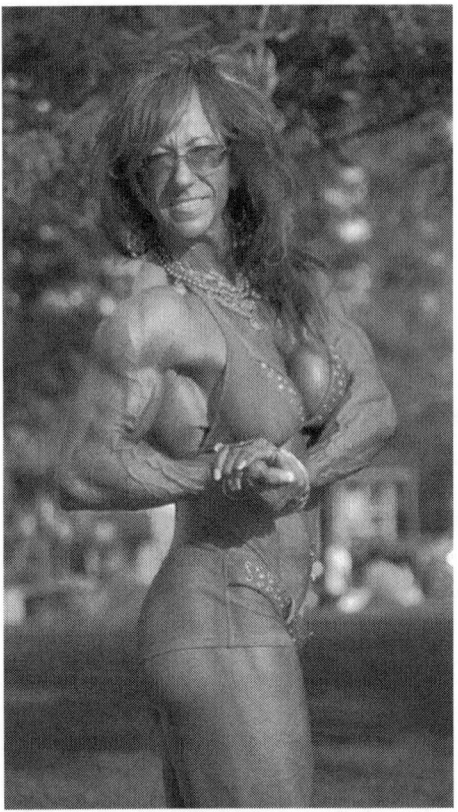

Cindy Johnson

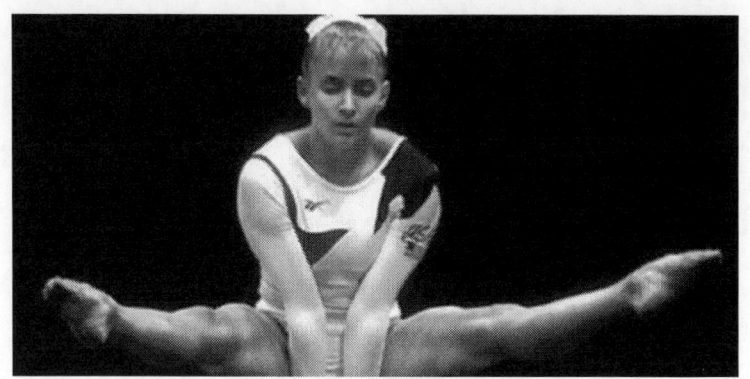

Shannon Miller

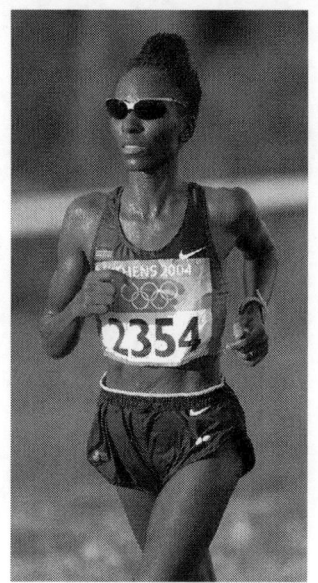

Catherine Ndereba

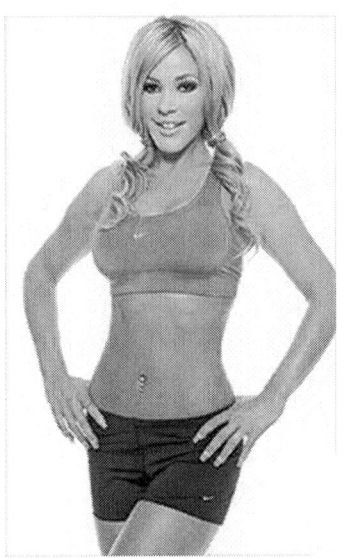

Chassidy Luke

Our gender and genetics should not be viewed as limitations but as assets to be maximized. I often ask my female clients if they have an ideal body image they'd like to achieve. What type of physique would you like to have?

What athlete or famous person has the body you'd like? The answers range from muscled bodybuilder to the compact gymnast to the fitness model to leaned out runner. Not surprisingly, most often their answers match up to their genetics. My answer to them is; OK, then we'll train like you want to look.

So what's the best way to train and are there bodyweight exercises that are better for women? If you don't' want to be sport-specific but just want to be fit, lean and strong, then a growing body of research indicates that multi-joint exercises performed in short time bursts (30-60 Sec) with short rest periods (15-30 sec) are superior for accelerating the muscle building and fat burning functions of the metabolism rather than lifting weights and counting repetitons.

This form of exercise is called High-Intensity Interval Training; HIIT. **You can train this way just using your bodyweight to provide the**

stimulus necessary for stimulating the muscle building functions within your genetic and gender defined metabolism.

At Fit4UrLife, the majority of our programs are based on the principles of High-Intensity Interval Training. This training is the fusion of anaerobic/strength exercises with aerobic/cardio exercises.

The workouts are time-based bouts of exercise; 20-90 sec of near maximal anaerobic/strength effort followed by a short rest period: 10-45 secs. Because of the intensity of this type of workout, we limit the workouts to 30-45 mins.

We do these exercises with and without weights. This is especially useful when we go to a clients home where they may not have exercise equipment available and where we are limited to what kind of weights we have available.

A web search on High-Intensity Interval Training will yield lots of information and links to the research so instead of boring you with lots of academic stuff, let's establish some useful principles you can apply starting today to enable you to get fit and build strong muscles without weights.

In a well-designed HIIT program exercises are grouped using supersets, circuits, complexes and other arrangements. In this high intensity/workload style of training, we never perform the same workout twice because we want to avoid having the muscles adapt. We are also just as disciplined about the rest periods as we are about the work periods.

Research has shown that this form of training is not only superior for building muscle and strength, but also provides great cardiovasular benefits and burns body fat, especially that troublesome belly fat.

The best feature is that many of these exercise just use bodyweight or can be augmented with bodyweight training aids like the TRX Suspension System, Perfect Push-Up, and Perfect Pull-Up, (1).

I have been using HIIT-based principles in my personal fitness program for the last 2-3 years and the results I've achieved are excellent. I have always been a big muscular guy to start with but since adopting HIIT principles, I have lost body fat (especially belly fat) and gained more definition and vascularity along with greater strength and endurance for my favorite sports like rowing, cycling, and cross-country skiing.

I particularly favor push-ups, pull-ups, squats, lunges, stair climbers and crunches combined with a variety of total body movements like side-to-side skater hops and box jumps; all performed with bodyweight and or assistive apparatus like the TRX Suspension System, the Perfect Push-Up, and Perfect Pull-Up. I also use many of the HIIT techniques and exercises I will be describing with my personal training clients when I go to their homes.

My wife and I do HIIT style classes at our local gym 2-3 times per week. These classes are taught by female instructors, use a mix of bodyweight and light dumbbells, and are absolutely fantastic. At our gym, they are listed as "Body Sculpting w/abs".
Other gyms might call them "Boot Camp" or "Hi-Intensity". Just make sure the instructors follow the principles I will outline in this chapter.

(1),We are not paid to endorse these products. We mention them because they are excellent products for using bodyweight to build muscle.

HIIT Principles

HIIT Principle 1: Focus on shoulders and hips. Why? Because the muscles in these areas are the most metabolically active muscle groups in the body and, when stimulated using multi-joint exercise in conjunction with the other HIIT principles, can provide maximal muscle building and fat burning metabolic stimulation.

Multi-joint exercises have also been shown to produce larger increases of anabolic (muscle building) hormones compared with single-joint exercises,(2). This is good news for both men and women because men get bigger muscles and women get stronger and more shapely muscles. These factors also improve overall health and fitness.

HIIT Principle 2: Volume and Time. To achieve the most effective muscle stimulating results we need to combine time with volume of work. There are four commonly used volume/time training methods:

1. Volume-specific intervals
2. Time-specific intervals
3. Timed volume-specific intervals
4. Density training

We'll discuss each one and how they stack up to HIIT.

1. Volume-specific intervals: This uses a fixed number of sets/reps or the movement to a specific fixed distance. For example, perform 15 pushups followed by 60 seconds of rest for 3 sets. For a distance, run a 440 yard (1 lap around a standard track) followed by a 220 yard walk/recovery. *These is pretty much how most people train and quite frankly, is probably the least effective way to effectively build muscle and lose fat.* The body quickly adapts to this style of training and it just does not provide enough metabolic stimuli to sustain muscle growth. However, if your goal is to build strength or endurance, then this method is most useful. Olympic and powerlifters use this technique almost exclusively. In fact, they often calculate their workouts in terms of poundage (volume) lifted.

When I was a competitive powerlifter, I would often gauge my training in terms of tonnage (volume). For example, when I did a squat workout, I'd add up all the poundage's used in each set and multiply by the reps (not counting warm-ups). For example, in a typical squat workout I'd do 6 sets of squats starting with 315 Lbs. for 10 reps for the first set; that would be 315x10 = 3,150 Lbs.

I'd pyramid up from there, adding up the poundsxreps totals. It is also the same for runners/cyclist only they calculate in terms of distance. Time is a secondary factor: how many tons did I lift today or how many miles did I run or ride this week?

(2),Hansen, S., et al. 2001. The effect of short-term strength training on human skeletal muscle: The importance of physiologically elevated hormone levels. Scandinavian Journal of Medicine & Science in Sports, 11 (6), 347–54.

2. Time-specific intervals: This alternates between a timed work period and a rest period for a certain number of rounds. One of the most popular time-specific interval techniques is the Tabata protocol, (3),where you work for 20-seconds followed by a rest of 10-seconds. It is most often done in aerobic classes like indoor cycling but I've also used it in our HIIT programs. For example, we do 2-second pushups (1 second down, 1 second up) for 20-seconds followed by 10-seconds of rest (remaining in the starting or plank position).

   Three rounds is one set and at 90-seconds will leave you pumped and breathing hard. If you follow immediately with a transition to lower body (hips/glutes/legs) exercise like lunges at 20/10 for three rounds, then you have one HIIT cycle based on the Tabata protocol.

3. Timed volume-specific intervals: This adds time to the volume-specific work and so requires the performance of a fixed number of reps or distance within a fixed time. For example, perform 15 pushups followed by 15 lunges in one minute. Run that 440 lap with a goal to finish in 2:30.

   If you finish in 2 minutes then you have 30-seconds to rest before the next 440. The faster you complete the exercises, the more rest time you will have. Man, talk about motivation! Doing a certain number of timed intervals would be a cycle.

4. Density training: This involves performing the maximum number of reps for time. This is probably the toughest protocol because you need an all out effort. For example, perform as many pushups, squats, burpees, (or combinations) etc., for 2 minutes with no rest or resting only as needed.

One of my favorites is to do 10 box squats with 10 side-to-side skater hops every 30-second for 3 minutes (6 sets). Simple, no equipment and builds muscle, power and endurance in the legs, glutes, and hips. It's a killer!

HIIT Principle 3: Time under tension. As discussed earlier, lots of research has shown that doing multiple sets of 8-15 reps that take 30-60 seconds to complete provides the greatest metabolic muscle-building stimulus. When done with short rest intervals, you are training in the hypertrophy (lactic acid) zone. Lactic acid is a byproduct of the Anaerobic-Glycolytic energy system, with the lactic acid produced as a byproduct of glycogen breakdown.

Bodybuilders have used this lactic acid style of training for years, and many world-class athletes have found that this style of training allows them to compete at higher levels of intensity because their bodies adapt to the higher levels of lactic acid. Some elite athletes like Olympic swimmer Michael Phelps appear to be gifted with certain genetic factors that either don't produce high levels of lactic acid, or allow their bodies to manage high levels of lactic acid while continuing to perform with minimal fatigue.

(3),The term comes from the name of Japanese scientist Izumi Tabata who, in a 1994 study, demonstrated that his 20-second work/10-second rest protocol showed improvements in both anaerobic and aerobic systems over traditional volume specific training. Available at:

Keeping the muscles under tension is the best way to encourage the body to produce the hormonal responses required to build muscle. Under tension can be thought of as a continuum: from very slow reps to fast, continuous reps for a short time periods. I never go over 90-seconds on any exercise or combination of exercises and most of the times remain in the 30-60 seconds range.

HIIT Principle 4: Work/Rest Energy Management. According to the National Strength and Conditioning Association (NSCA), growth hormone is one of the most effective muscle building and fat burning hormones produced by the body as a result of intense exercise followed by short rest periods lasting no more than 60 seconds.

A quick review of the body's energy systems can help us understand and appreciate why intense exercise followed by short rest periods is so effective. The body has two energy systems: aerobic and anaerobic. Based on the training intensity and time, one may be used more than the other may.

The anaerobic energy system produces energy using creatine-phosphogen stored in the muscles without using oxygen but can only do so for 10-20 seconds to produce maximal bursts of strength and power.

The anaerobic-glycolytic system also produces energy without using oxygen but can do so by breaking down carbs circulating in the blood (glycolysis).

The byproduct of this glycogen breakdown is lactic acid and the energy can produce strength and power for 30-60 seconds. Your aerobic system uses oxygen along with carbs and stored fat (oxidative phosphorylation) to sustain lower levels of intensity for activity lasting longer periods.

Each of these systems has a specific work to rest interval and you guessed it, HIIT targets the anaerobic-glycolytic system most effectively. I have found that the 20/10 Tabata protocol can scale up within that range: 30 work/15 rest and 60 work/30 rest.

According to recent studies, (4),short rest periods following intense effort may cause a significant amount of metabolic stress, which is now believed to be a potent stimulator for muscle and strength building.

(4),Schoenfeld, B.J. 2011. *The use of specialized training techniques to maximize muscle hypertrophy. Strength and Conditioning Journal, 33 (4), 60–65.*

Exercising HIIT style for women

So now that we've got these HIIT principles in mind, let's turn to the actual exercises starting with the exercise that many fitness experts consider the best all-around bodyweight exercise: the squat. You do squats every time you sit down or get up from a chair.

The squat not only involves the leg and buttock muscles (hip joint) but also the trunk (core) muscles as stabilizers; some of the largest, strongest, and most metabolically active muscles in the body. Performed with bodyweight and at various speeds and foot placement patterns, it can also produce significant cardiovascular benefits and, as those big muscles work, burn lots of fat.

For my female clients I like to use lunges. They are a nice alternative to the squat and can be done in a variety of foot placement styles. They really target the glutes, which is one area where just about every woman wants to improve and, which many of my female clients want to specifically target. I often alternate the two: a squat followed by a lunge.

I do not want to waste time and space describing how to perform squats and lunges. Many web sites have plenty of videos that show how to properly perform these exercises. What I want to emphasize here is HIIT Muscle Building Principles, especially principle 1: squats combined with upper body exercise and performed using the other HIIT principles will maximize metabolic stimulation for building muscle, strength, and fat loss.

Speaking of upper body exercises, it is the push up that is the upper body equivalent to the squat. The push up involves all the major muscles of the shoulder girdle, arms, and the core muscles for stabilization. I was one of the few guys in the Army (Ranger/Airborne) that really enjoyed the physical training and especially doing push ups. I can do them all day long and often do.

However, for women, I have to be careful because I don't want to overdo the push up exercise. Women generally do not possess the upper body strength of men, and so modifications are necessary. For a woman who is just starting out, the wall push-up is best.

- Wall push-up: Stand with your feet shoulder width apart facing a wall. Step back about arms length. Raise your arms up horizontal and place your hands flat against the wall with your arms straight out and at the same height and slightly wider than your shoulders. Allow your body to slowly "lower" toward the wall, keeping your back straight and head up, until your upper arm is at a 90-degree angle from your lower arm. Press yourself back to the straight arm starting point. Do as many of these as you can while keeping good form. Over time, try to speed up and do more repetitions.

The next level of effort is the modified (or assisted) push up.

- Modified Push-Up: You assume the normal push up position or "plank", then lower your knees to the floor while keeping your arms straight and slightly wider than your shoulders. You then perform the push up by lowering your upper body toward the floor until your upper arm is at a 90-degree angle to your lower arm. Push yourself back up to the starting position. Doing these slowly and in a controlled way will help build your strength which will eventually allow you to do the regular push-up.

Progress from the wall to the modified and then to the regular push-up. Again, lots of web sites have excellent examples of how to do a push-up and its many variations and modifications.

One progression I have taught in moving from the modified to the full push-up is the use of eccentric reps (negatives) and isometrics. For example, an eccentric (negative) rep would be performed like this:

- Start in the plank position and slowly lower yourself down until your elbow is at a 90-degree angle. Then drop down to your knees and press yourself back up – the second half of the modified push-up. Repeat for 5 reps.
- An isometric rep would be done like this: Start out in the plank position and lower yourself about ¾ of the way down – then pause and hold for a count of 10 – or as much as you can hold it. Drop to your knees and press yourself back up and repeat for 5 reps.

Isometrics and negatives are great strength builders but they create lots of delayed onset muscle soreness, so make sure you have some analgesics on hand to take for the discomfort.

Push-ups and squats/lunges are the two core exercises for building muscles without using weights. A simple combination of different types of squats alternated with different styles of push-ups done for multiple sets using the HIIT principles will yield tremendous results.

We don't want to forget the abs so finish with mountain climbers and leg lifts, and side-to-side crunches to get the obliques. You can do a very simple push-up/squat-lunge and ab workout in about 20 minutes to stimulate the metabolic muscle building and fat loss functions very effectively. When traveling, I often perform this type of workout in my hotel room.

Another one of my favorite upper body exercises is the pull up. However, it is hard for a woman to perform using bodyweight unless she has built a base of upper body strength and many women have not developed this strength base. However, you can do pull-ups if you work at it.

<u>Just because you're a woman doesn't mean you can't do pull-ups so you're not off the hook ladies!</u>

One major point about doing pull-ups: Handgrip position is key. There are two basic positions: Forward grip (palms facing away from you) and reverse (curl) grip (palms facing you). (Technically, the reverse grip is a chin and the forward grip is a pull-up). The forward grip involves the upper back muscles more and is much harder for women to perform.

The reverse (curl) grip is slightly easier as you get more bicep involvement. I recommend starting out with the reverse grip and once you're able to do several reps, change to training with the forward grip.

Female gymnasts and bodybuilders do them all the time, you just need to build your upper body strength through discipline and training.

Flash forward into the future: You walk into the gym, stroll past all the muscle heads and as their eyes follow you (probably because you've been doing lots of lunges and squats), suddenly you jump up and start cranking out chins! Or think about how you'll look in that slinky black dress with the low cut back. You betcha!

There are three ways to build your upper body strength: assisted (cheater) reps, eccentric (negatives) or isometrics (like we discussed for push-ups).

- Assisted (cheater) reps: Have your training partner lift you into position and then assist you by lifting you up as you perform the pull-ups. The partner can grab you at the waist, or you can bend your legs back and they can hold your shins and assist you from there.

- Eccentric (negatives): Jump up, or have your training partner lift you up and grab the bar as you would be in the full pull up or ending position. Then slowly lower yourself down to the starting position in a controlled manner. Repeat for 4-5 reps.

- Isometrics: Again, jump up or have your training partner assist you into a position where you are a little more than half way up. Hold that position for as long as you can up to 10-seconds. Then slowly lower yourself down. Repeat 4-5 times.

It is also difficult to perform if you don't have access to some structure that can allow you to do pull ups. I've tried to use the pull up bars that fit in a doorway, but don't feel comfortable with them. So I often go to public parks with my Perfect Pull Up handles, find some monkey bars or a swing set and do them there.

Where to work out?

Because you don't need weights or machines, you can work out using these principles just about anywhere: Your bedroom, garage, back yard, deck, park, hotel room (no excuses if you are on vacation), etc. Many fitness clubs, gyms, and personal trainers now offer HIIT style group exercises classes.

Recently the "boot camp" style has become quite popular. I've attended several and found that some instructors don't understand the principles I've outlined here and so don't incorporate them in their boot camps, so it's caveat emptor. Remember, it's your workout.

There are also popular videos like Tony Horton's P90X® and others. A web search on "HIIT workouts" will net you lots of videos and workouts. If you hire a personal trainer, make sure that they understand how to implement the HIIT principles for your training program. It's your money, so get your money's worth!

Some words about Nutrition for Building Muscle

As mentioned in the introduction, the only two muscle building factors we can control are the resistance exercise stimulus and nutritional intake. Concerning nutrition, I try to get everything I need from my whole foods diet.

I stay away from sodium, sugar, and gluten as much as possible and focus on chicken, fish, lean beef and eggs as main protein source. The only dairy we consume is non-fat Greek yogurt per the Dukan diet. My wife and I follow a dietary pattern based on the Dukan diet maintenance plan and it has given us excellent muscle building and fat reduction results.

In addition to my diet, I take protein shakes made from high quality whey protein. I try to get at least 0.5 gram of protein per pound of bodyweight per day.

I have seen recommendations that vary from a third of an ounce per pound of bodyweight all the way up to 2 grams per pound of bodyweight but for my body, genetics, and metabolism, 0.5g/Lb. of bodyweight per day works great.

One thing I have observed is that many women don't get enough high quality protein in their diet. Just observe at a restaurant where the man orders the tuna fish sandwich and the woman orders the salad with a few small pieces of chicken.

Ladies, if you're gonna train HIIT style, then you need to make sure you're taking in enough quality protein to support muscoe building and recovery. You'll need to experiment to see what is enough because everyone is different. When I started taking in too much, I started gaining some belly fat. That's how I knew.

I have clients that follow Weight Watchers or other programs and are getting good results. Other clients have gone to Registered Dieticians and received personalized diet counseling.

These diets and programs work if you stay with the programs – especially the maintenance phase. Many people go on them, lose their weight, and then go off the diet instead of doing the maintenance.

All that discipline to lose the weight and then no discipline to stick with the most important part of any diet program: the maintenance. That's how they gain their weight back and enter the yo-yo dieting cycle. It's not rocket surgery but it does require behavioral change, dedication, and discipline.

Any discussion of nutrition for building muscle must also address supplementation. Nutritional supplementation is a multi-billion dollar a year industry.

There is a growing body of clinical research on multivitamins, antioxidants, fish oil, etc., that show these substances produce minimal to no results.

For example, an *American Medical Association Journal* article from last year compared cancer mortality rates for people who had taken multivitamins to those who did not.

The results showed that those who took multivitamins had a slightly lower risk of cancer. Other studies on cardiovascular disease show no difference at all. Similar clinical study results are being experienced for antioxidants, fish oil, etc.

I've contributed thousands of dollars to it over the years myself and I can tell you it has been largely a waste of money. Everyone's genetics and thus his or her metabolisms are different. I've had clients and friends that swear by a certain supplement but when I took it, I got little to no results.

However, I still keep experimenting because I want to be able to advise my clients appropriately. In fact, the only supplement I take regularly is Chia Seed. Yes, that's right Chia Seed – like the Chia Pet plants as seen on TV.

They are a natural supplement that gives me a great burst of energy for a couple of hours but without the exhausted let down often experienced by synthetic energy boosters.

I first learned about Chia in Christopher McDougall's book *Born to Run*. In the book, McDougall describes the almost superhuman ability of Mexico's Tarahumara Indians for running long distances without stopping, or chasing deer until the deer becomes exhausted and can't run anymore.

The Tarahumara combine Chia with *Pinole*, a type of corn that is roasted and ground into cornmeal. They can run for days just sustaining themselves on these two substances along with drinking water from streams. Chia works for me and it's inexpensive.

If you feel you need to do supplements and can afford the cost, then do them. I do.

Muscle Building and Drugs

We've all seen the roid monsters in the gym and in various magazines. These guys and some gals are huge and ripped and they all claim that they are natural.

Baloney! We've seen the scandals of famous athletes (male and female) who have taken performance-enhancing substances. I can tell you for a fact that, while they might have good genetics that favor adding muscle mass, no one can add that kind of freaky mass without the help of anabolic steroids.

128

When I was a powerlifter in my late 20's, I experimented with anabolic steroids. At 6"1", I put on 40-pounds in a year – I got huge.

My bench press went from 335 to 475+. My squat and deadlift were even better. I was regularly totaling over 1800 lbs. in competitions and my goal was to break 2000 at a body weight of 260.

My training partner and I were "stacking" 2 different veterinary steroids; steroids that were not developed for human consumption. We were consuming thousands of calories per day.

A dozen scrambled eggs for breakfast each day. Whole roasted chickens for lunch and 2-3 rib eye steaks a piece for dinner. However, the side effects were noticeable and drastic and I soon had to stop or risk permanent damage to my physical and mental health.

Ladies, do not go down this path. Some have and it is a path to certain destruction of your body and maybe even your life. I've seen it first hand.

The temporary gains just aren't worth the risk. If you think they are then you need psychological help. I know, I've stared down that rabbit hole and didn't like what I saw.

Hormone Replacement Therapy

I want to finish the chapter by discussing the growing trend of hormone replacement therapy. As men age, their natural ability to produce the metabolic muscle building hormone testosterone decreases. In women, estrogen and progesterone also decrease with age and drop off even more with menopause.

The results are diminished sex drive, depression, fatigue, and loss of muscle mass. In men, the "Lo-T" problem can also result in testicular atrophy and even an increased chance of having heart disease.

Again, there are many expensive supplements on the market that claim to raise T-levels, but the most effective way is to seek bio-identical replacement therapy from a qualified medical professional.

When I turned 60 I started losing strength and endurance, could not recover adequately between workouts, started gaining fat no matter how I adjusted my diet, and was experiencing bouts of depression along with decreased libido. Over time, it got worse no matter what I did. In short, I felt like I was turning into an old man.

My wife, also a life long athlete, was experiencing similar problems and, even though she is several years younger, she had gone through menopause. She began bio-identical hormone replacement therapy and the results she experienced were phenomenal. I couldn't keep up with her!

Based on her results, I began bio-identical testosterone therapy about a year and-a-half ago and it has been incredible. I had begun experiencing all the symptoms and my T-levels were very low at the start.

However, there was still so much left to do and so many adventures to be had – so much more life to be lived with my beautiful wife!

I now feel tremendous and all the original symptoms are gone. I'm 63 and perform in the gym, on the bike and in the bedroom as if I was half that age. Ladies, you owe it to yourself to investigate this therapy. It isn't cheap but if you want to keep enjoying life as you age and not become a wobbly old woman, then check into this therapy.

About Buck Nimz

Fit4UrLife

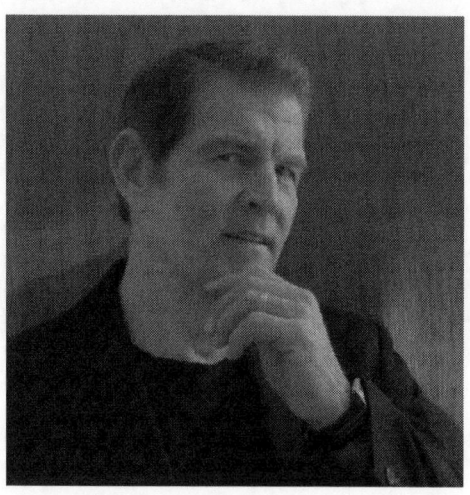

I've been doing personal training and strength coaching for over 20-years. My wife, Cynthia, is a Doctor of Physical Therapy and a certification specialist for the Aerobics and Fitness Association of America (AFAA). We recently started Fit4UrLife as a second career and as a vehicle for bringing new and innovative ideas to the fitness market and to our clients.

Many people we talk to have developed a negative impression of personal trainers because they watch the TV shows where grossly obese people are sweating profusely, huffing and puffing, falling off treadmills, collapsing in total exhaustion, and even vomiting.

All the while, the trainer is screaming at them like a drill sergeant. That image of personal trainers is a lot more pervasive than many realize and it is just flat out wrong. It makes me angry! Our approach to personal training is unique in several ways. For example, I train with many of our clients as if I was their training partner.

Many personal trainers just stand there and tell the client what to do and count the reps; they never break a sweat. I consider that more coaching than training. We have a different service model.

As a life long athlete, I had training partners. We were committed to our training and encouraged each other to excel. We knew that the other partner was there at the gym waiting for us so we didn't want to let them down. I want to be my client's partner. I want them to have the experience of having a partner who is committed to their success.

I want to be sweating and huffing and puffing right next to them because it provides the kind of encouragement and reinforcement they need. They can see that I'm investing my time and energy in getting them to reach their goals. Our services are not cheap, so we owe our clients maximum results for their investment.

That means I often get 3-4 workouts a day. When I tell other trainers this, they think I'm crazy. But I know my body and how to pace myself. I also know how to recover and when to back off and slip into the coaching mode.

I'm experienced in all different populations: from the deconditioned businessman to the elite athlete, high school to older adults; pregnant women and post-partum. I've trained teams and individual competitive athletes. I've recently begun focusing on the tactical athlete and taking advantage of my military experience. Our goal: Get you Fit 4 Ur Life, whatever life you want.

Questions or comments? Email buck.nimz@gmail.com. Our Fit4UrLife web page will be up soon.

CHAPTER 6

Elyssa Bulthuis

Simple Moves for a Smoking Hot Body

Whether you're looking just to tone or to build larger muscles, both can be obtained through body weight training. Exercises using only your body weight as resistance are an effective and functional way to train your body.

One of the best reasons to train this way is that you are much less likely to injure yourself than when training with heavy weights, yet you can see much of the same results. From squats to pull ups, body weight training is appropriate for everyone -- and it's free!

Body weight training eliminates:
- Gym memberships
- Home gym equipment
- Tricky choreography
- Excuses to not exercise when traveling
- Risks of many typical workout injuries
- Bulking up
- Wasted time driving to and from the gym

Body weight training assures that you are not lifting too much weight for you! You simply will not be able to complete the exercise if it's not appropriate for you AT THIS TIME. Unlike a machine that assists with part of the weight bearing and may convince you to lift more than you should resulting in muscle injuries, your body weight is never too much for you to move or lift.

Over time, you will definitely build the strength to do, for example, a pull up, even though your first efforts may fail you. Don't worry! We can modify the exercise to build those muscles.

Furthermore, body weight training packs a serious cardio punch.

By interspersing cardio movements between your weight bearing exercises, you will become a calorie inferno! Another benefit is the ease of moving between exercises is as you don't have to waste time changing weights or waiting for machines to open up at the gym which will cause your heart rate to slow down when you don't want it to do so.

What You'll Need:

While you won't need any expensive equipment, there are some items you may want to purchase to make your workouts efficient.

- A workout mat - getting rug burns or sliding on floor surfaces is painful and dangerous. A mat also creates a safe barrier between you and (the god-knows-what people have walked in on the bottom of their shoes) bacteria on the floor.

- A timer or clock with a second hand - circuit training and high intensity interval training require timers. If you have a smart phone you are already set with the clock function. You can also download FREE interval timers and Tabata timers to keep the counting simple.

- Good cross training shoes.

- A towel and water bottle

- A fun option is a dry erase board or a chalkboard to write your workout on. It makes going through your workout easier to keep of track of and is great motivation as you see yourself progress in the session. You can even post your personal best times or reps to keep you challenging yourself.

Before you begin this or any other workout, be sure to have medical clearance.

What you'll also require:

- Commitment
- Drive
- Determination
- Quantifiable goals

I'm assuming that if you are focusing on a body weight exercise plan, you aren't heading to the gym to do this workout! Working out alone at home takes considerable **commitment and drive**.

You will need to schedule your work out time and put it on your calendar as a "nothing gets in the way of my workout time" activity.

Just like you wouldn't schedule a business call during your dentist appointment or agree to babysit someone else's child on a day that your own kids are with the grandparents, consider your workout time as sacrosanct -- nothing else can be scheduled during that time which includes business meetings or calls, watching TV, or going out with friends.

Being disciplined is the first step in reaching your goals. This requires your **determination** to make exercise a natural part of your day like brushing your teeth (please tell me you do this daily!).

"The pain of discipline is far less than the pain of regret."
—Sarah Bombell

Goals and Results
Nothing makes you quit working out like not seeing results. But what results are you looking for? If you say your goal of working out is to "get healthy" or "get stronger," what the heck does that mean?

Your goals need to be quantifiable and measurable. For example:

"After 4 weeks of exercise, I will be able to perform 5 more push ups than I can today."
 "I will be able to do 20 burpees in 1 minute after 6 weeks."

"After 6 weeks of cardio workouts, I will be able to climb the stairs at my office without feeling winded."

"I will lose 2 lbs in 2 weeks."

All of these goals are precise and measurable. When you accomplish them, TELL EVERYONE and give yourself a prize! A manicure, an hour of reading or watching your favorite guilty pleasure TV show, a spa day. Whatever makes you feel special, do it.

But, what if you don't meet your goal? Ask yourself: Did I really commit to my workouts? Have I performed them at least 3 times a week? Have I pushed myself as hard as I needed to reach this goal?

Working out alone is challenging for most people. On our own, we don't push ourselves as hard as we would in a crowded class or with a trainer. However, you don't need either of these to up your commitment.

Here are 2 ideas to try. First, get a workout buddy. Knowing that someone is waiting on you to workout will get you to show up more regularly. It sounds trite, I know, but it works as long as the buddy is motivated to work out too!

Idea #2 will hit you in the pocket book. For the next 6 months, commit to working out 3 days per week for at least 30 minutes. Every time you miss, you must donate $10 (more or less depending on your income, but you have to make it hurt!) to a charity you despise. Are you a peace loving hippie?

Your money goes to the NRA! You are a staunch Republican? You donate to the Democratic National Convention. The more you make it hurt, the more impetus you have for showing up!

Let me know how this goes for you! Drop me an email at elyssa@getfitwithelyssa.com and I may feature your story in a future blog post.

Now, if you've been honest with your calorie intake and your workouts, you might need to go see a doctor to have your blood tested and get a physical to see what may be inhibiting your weight loss.

Get Moving!

The following are 3 body weight workouts showing 3 levels of difficulty for each exercise. You can choose to begin with Level 1 and progress to Level 3

OR

You can choose which exercise progression in order presented of the 10 exercises (e.g. marching high knees, jogging high knees, running high knees) best suits your level of fitness, and after three to four weeks, begin to challenge yourself with the next level.

Because in some areas you'll be able to do the more difficult exercise while in others you'll need to do the more basic move, these workouts will change and develop with you over time.

I've chosen exercises that you can easily look up online to get directions for how to perform them or I've given a brief description so you can get started right away.

Body weight 30 minute circuit - complete each exercise in a Level for 45 seconds then rest for 15 seconds and begin next exercise. Once you've completed all 10 exercises take a 1-minute break. Complete 3 rounds if possible.

Level 1
- Low impact jumping jack - keep one foot on the floor at all times

- Push-up against a wall or edge of a couch
- Squats
- Plank on knees
- Rear lunges alternating legs
- Marching high knees
- Hold a squat while throwing quick punches
- Crunches
- Side lying leg lifts right leg
- Side lying leg lifts left leg

Level 2

- Jumping jacks
- Push-ups on knees on floor
- 3 pulse squat then stand up
- Plank on hands and feet or forearms and feet
- Alternating rear lunges with 3 pulses before switching legs
- Jogging high knees
- Holding a plié squat throw 3 punches then hop up repeat
- Crunches lift with a three count raise and a one count lower
- Standing side leg lift with a squat
- Repeat other side

Level 3

- Jumping jacks
- Military push-ups
- Jump squats
- Plank on forearms and feet with alternating leg tap out to side
- Alternating jumping rear lunges
- Running high knees with arms reaching up and down overhead
- Holding a plié squat throw 3 punches then drop to floor jump legs back then hop back up to plié and repeat
- Crunch with alternating leg extension -- extending one leg up to ceiling, reach up to touch toes
- Curtsy squat with side leg lift
- Repeat other leg

To create more intensity to any of these circuits lengthen the work phase to 1 minute.

Tabatas:

Tabata training is quick and tough! Bodyweight exercises work great and you will be surprised at how challenging this high intensity interval is!

A timer is really helpful to keep track not only of the time but also how many intervals you've completed. There are free apps available for your smartphone or ipod that will tell you when to start and when to rest as well as count the rounds. It's easy to lose track in the heat of this workout!

You will do an exercise for 20 seconds of your all out effort followed by 10 seconds of recovery. You will repeat this for 4 minutes! Splitting the Tabata with two (or more) exercises makes it a tad easier and is a good way for beginners to approach this plan.

For example, in Level 1 you would perform Squats for 20 seconds, rest for 10 seconds, repeat the squats for 20 seconds, rest for 10 seconds, then do the rear lunges twice and return to the squats. Therefore, you will have completed 4 rounds of squats and 4 rounds of the lunges in the 4 minute time frame. Then move on to the push-ups and back extensions using the same time formula.

For Level 2, you will complete 1 exercise for the entire 4 minutes then move on to the next 3 exercises. And, in Level 3, you will complete 8 exercises for a total of 32 minutes. You might want to create your own Level 2.5 and add 2 exercises to your Tabata before going to the 8. Pace yourself!

Level 1

- Squats/alternating leg rear lunges
- Push-ups/prone back extensions
- Triceps dips/skaters
- Sit-ups/supine hip raises

Level 2

- Squats
- Push-ups
- Sit-ups

- Triceps dips

Level 3

- Jump squats
- Push ups
- Sit ups
- Triceps dips
- Slalom side jumps
- Side plank to side plank
- High knees
- Mountain climbers

Create your own circuits:

The following exercises should read as a menu for you to choose from for creating your own circuits or tabatas.

Start each of these workouts with a 5 minute warm up. For example jog or march in place, circle the arms, rhythmically stretch your back, do some hamstring curls, then step your legs apart, straighten them, and then reach your hand to the opposite foot alternating a few times to prepare for the workout.

End each workout with some static stretching. Interlace your hands in front of the body, turn the palms away from your body and then reach over head.

Keeping hands interlaced, bring arms shoulder height and round the upper back. Reach one arm over your head and stretch to the side and repeat with the other arm. Then bend over with straight legs and reach for your toes. Hold each stretch about 20-30 seconds breathing calmly and deeply.

Here are 5 ways you can use these exercises to keep your workouts dynamic and fresh:

Circuits: choose one exercise from each category; complete the exercise for 45 seconds to 1 minute, rest for 15 seconds and move to the next exercise. Complete all 8 exercises then rest for 1 minute. Complete 3 rounds

Cardio Strength Full Body Circuit: Choose 7 cardio moves and then insert 7 strength moves between them, one from each category. Use the same timing as above OR do Cardio for 2 minutes and strength training for 45 or 60 seconds.

Specialized Strength Upper or Lower Body Circuit: Choose only from the upper body or only from the lower body to "specialize" your circuit. Try doing the cardio moves for 2 minutes and the strength training for 45 seconds to 1 minute. Again, rest about 15-30 seconds between exercises. Complete the circuit 2-3 times.

For *Tabatas*, I suggest you alternate with upper then lower body moves as well. Don't be afraid to add in some cardio moves! Burpees, Skaters, Squat Jumps, High Knees or Box Jumps are great choices.

Don't choose more that 8 exercises for your tabatas and don't use more than 2 exercises from any one group as that will overly fatigue the muscles and could cause injury or at the very least you will be so sore you will never make that mistake twice.

HIITS: Pick 3 Cardio Moves and 1 exercise from each of the other groups. Perform 8-20 repetitions of three strength moves. Then do a 3 minute High Intensity Cardio Fartlek.

For example: squat for 30 seconds, then squat faster for 20 seconds, then jump squat as high and as fast as you can for 10 seconds. Repeat for 3 minutes.

So, take any of the cardio moves, perform them at pace that lightly challenges you for 30 seconds, really challenges you for 20 seconds, and then all out effort with your heart pounding out of your chest for 10 seconds repeating for 3 minutes. YOU CAN DO IT! Then repeat the first 3 strength moves for the 8-20 reps and repeat the HIIT.

Move on to the other 4 exercises and then repeat the HIITs between sets. You can use one cardio move for all of your HIITs on the upper body and then another for the HIITs between your lower body exercises or you can use 3 different cardio moves alternating throughout the workout.

Shoulders	Chest	Arms	Back
Arm Circles	Push ups	Punching (pick one or two): jabs, upper cuts, imaginary speed bag drill, hook	Low cobra lift and lower
Down Dog	Feet higher than shoulders push ups (feet on couch or bench)	Triceps dips - off the edge of a stair or bench	Prone "I" "T" & "Y" arm/upper back lifts
Down Dog Push Ups	Push off against wall/bench/floor - push your arms off the surface and land lightly with bent elbows	Walking push ups - side to side or forward and back	Superman back extensions – legs remain on floor upper body lifts and lowers

143

Inverted Down Dog with feet on wall or chair	Feet on the wall even with shoulders push up	Crawl outs/inch worms - start standing, bend over, walk hands out to top of push up then walk hands back to feet and stand up	Superman both -- arms and legs lift and lower
Dolphin pose (Down dog but with your forearms on the ground not just your hands) http://www.yogajournal.com/poses/2462	Push ups with one hand on a raised platform (phone book duck taped shut?!)	Plank ups - from high plank, lower on to your elbows then straighten arms back to high plank	Prone swimming-- flutter arms or breast stroke
Dolphin on wall (Forearms on the ground, feet on wall at hip height)		Triceps push ups	Standing on one leg lean forward bringing other leg even with shoulder height balance in airplane position and create swimming motion with arms

Shoulders	Chest	Arms	Back
Dolphin near wall (Legs extended to sky, heels resting on wall)			Prone Superman Lift chest twist and shoulder look over shoulder, repeat looking over other shoulder
Handstand near wall			
Side plank	TRX & Pull Up Bar	TRX & Pull Up Bar	TRX & Pull Up Bar

Legs	Gluteals	Core	Cardio Moves
Forward Lunges	Squats	Standing knee to elbow twist	Shuffles
Side Lunges	Squats with forward kicks	In chair pose, reach opposite elbow to knee, return to center repeat	Skaters
Rear Lunges	Squats with side kicks	Supine crunches	Burpees
Diagonal Lunges	Sumo Squats	Plank holds	Jump squats
Walking Lunges	Curtsy Squats	Plank touch knee to elbow	Jump rope (real or imaginary)
Lunges with balance - hold knee up in front of chest after lunge	Plié squats	Plank touch knee to opposite elbow	High knees
Lunges with hop changing forward leg	Squats with rear kicks	Side plank lift and lower hip to floor	Jog in place

Legs	Gluteals	Core	Cardio Moves
Quadruped (Hands and knees position) Lift leg to hip height then bend and straighten leg	Lunges - in every direction	Boat Pose	Wide leg football fast feet
Side Lying leg lifts, leg circles	Supine bent knee hip raises with feet and knees about 5" apart - variation one leg lifts to sky and remains raised through set	Criss cross bicycle crunches	Running stairs

Inner thigh - side lying bend top knee place foot on floor behind bottom leg then lift bottom leg to height of back knee then lower	Supine bent knee hip raises with feet and knees touching	Prone opposite arm & leg lifts	Hopping forward and back or side to side
Squats	Supine bent knee hip raises with feet touching and knees apart	Prone lift both arms and both legs lift at same time	Jumping up on a bench or step
	Quadruped (table pose) rear leg lifts- straight or bent knee	From prone swim with arms and legs breast stroke or flutter arms	Mountain Climbers standing or prone

Playing with time and intensity and using a variety of moves will keep your sessions interesting, challenging, and productive. If 45 or 60 second intervals are too tough to start with, begin with 30 seconds and rest for 30 seconds or even a minute between sets.

It takes time to build endurance and strength so don't be hard on yourself when you first begin. It's better to be able to finish and be successful with what you've chosen than to feel defeated every time you try.

You can create your own 15, 30, 45 or 60 minute workouts from these circuits (except the Tabatas - no more than 30 minutes with those) by the amount of exercises you choose and the amount of repetitions of the circuit. You may only want to do a circuit one time through the first few days out and then build up to two rounds etc.

When you are ready for more challenges, you can invest in some basic equipment to shake your workout up again.

Basic Equipment:

Here are some basic pieces of equipment that will enhance your workouts but are NOT necessary for the workouts I've included in this chapter. These are great additions as you improve your strength and will add interest and variety to your routines.

Chin Up Bar

A chin up bar in your doorway adds the possibility for increasing your upper body strength and adding more basic exercises to your routine.

When you first start using a bar, begin with negative chin ups and pull ups. Use a chair or step stool to get your chin higher than the bar and then lower your body as slowly as possible. Of course starting out on the bar is pretty darn tough.

The negative, or lowering, portion is however attainable for the moderately fit woman and will prepare you for the full move. Another way to make the pull up and chin up easier is to use an elastic exercise band around the bar. Create a loop that you can place your foot into.

This will support a portion of your weight. Use the least amount of leg strength as possible and work your upper body as much as possible.

This will improve your latissimus dorsi muscles on your sides and back. Women's backs typically are quite weak and our ability to lift our own body weight is almost unheard of.

Training with a pull up bar will improve your posture, strengthen your back and you'll notice you carry yourself better when your back is strong. The chin up and pull up will also give you killer arms with tons of definition.

Bench
Nothing fancy here, just something you can step up onto that is sturdy. If you have an old Step-Aerobics bench, that will work, or you can step up onto a high stair, strong chair, or old fashioned bench. Make sure it is strong enough to support your weight and is stable!

Now you can add box jumps to your cardio/leg workouts. Begin with a height slightly lower than your knees and practice jumping up and down off the bench working your way up to 1 minute of non-stop jumping. Then begin to raise the platform by 2" or so. Go as high as you feel safe doing so!

TRX
TRX is suspension training that uses your body weight against angles to make progressions and regressions of exercises easier.

A suspension trainer can make push ups more accessible by raising the angle but adds more core work by requiring stabilization due to the imbalance created by the straps.

A TRX can move you from nearly completely upright push ups against the wall feel to facilitating an inverted handstand push up with your feet instead of your hands in the cradles.

This one piece of equipment (which travels nicely) will add more diversity and challenges to your body weight training and can be used by beginners and experts alike. However, it costs around $200.

If you've tried these workouts you know that simple does not mean easy! Returning to basic movements while using just your body weight and a few pieces of equipment will get you to a strong, toned, sleek, smoking hot body in no time at all.

About Elyssa Bulthuis

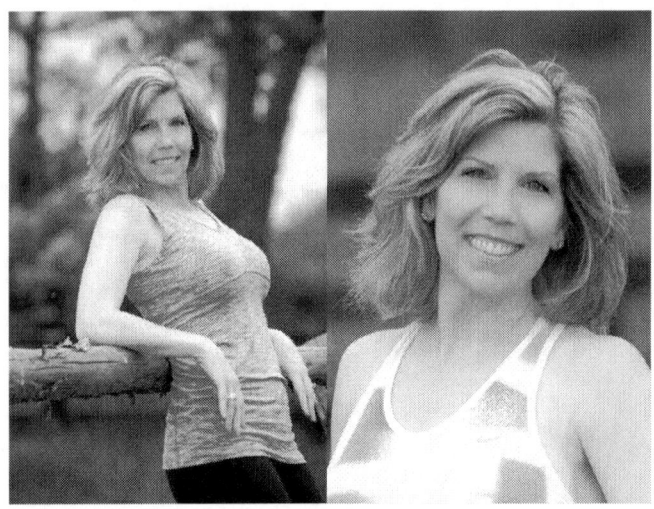

I've been a group fitness and yoga instructor since 1998. I hold certifications with AFAA for Group Instruction, with Moksha Yoga Chicago, and with ACSM as a Personal Trainer.

A few years ago, I traveled to India to study yoga at the Krishnamacharya Yoga Mandiram in Chennai where I deepened my knowledge of meditation and asana practice. I include yoga practices for most of my personal training clients as I believe flexibility is equally important to strength.

This year I completed a Tough Mudder and my first mini-triathlon. Besides fitness, I hold an MA in English and am a sometimes Adjunct at the University of St. Francis in Joliet, IL as well as a beekeeper at our horse farm in Frankfort, IL.

You can connect with me at my website www.getfitwithelyssa.com and on Facebook at **http://www.facebook.com/getfitwithelyssa** or email me at elyssa@getfitwithelyssa.com

Would You Be Willing To Leave A Review?

If you would consider writing a review of this book on Amazon, I would very much appreciate it. The feedback I receive from readers will be helpful as I develop updates to this book and create other related books.

To write a review of this book, just type 'Andy Charalambous' in the Amazon search bar and click on reviews.

If you have any comments or questions regarding anything to do with this book then please don't hesitate to send me an email at fitscribbler@gmail.com

Thank you so much,

Andy Charalambous

Recommended Related Books

More Books you may like by Andy Charalambous

Just type 'Andy Charalambous' in the Amazon search bar to see all of his latest books:

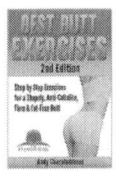 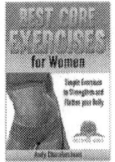 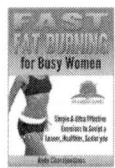 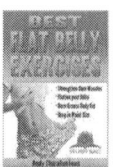 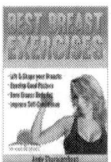

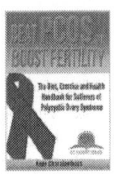 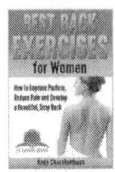 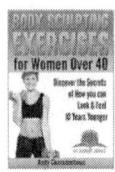 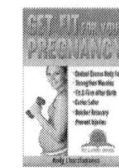 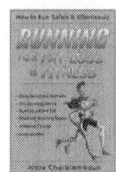

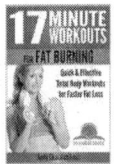 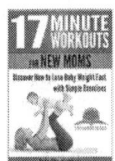 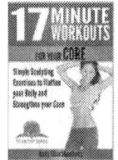 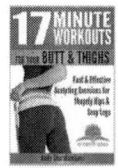 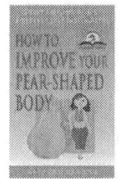

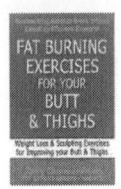 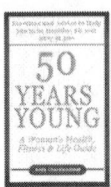 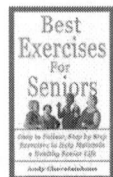 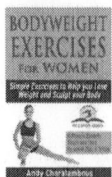 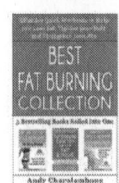

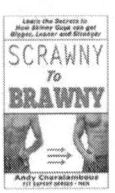 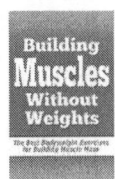 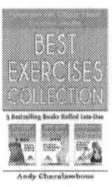 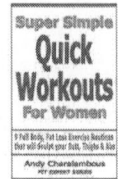

About the Author

Andy Charalambous

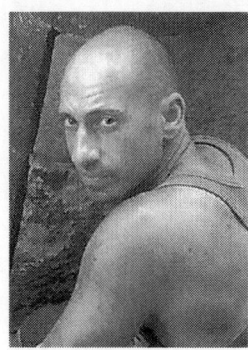

Andy Charalambous was born in London, England and has worked in a number of well-known health clubs and gyms as a fitness instructor, personal trainer and masseur.

He is not your average trainer! He has taken on fat loss experiments where he has gained weight in order to document how he will eventually lose the weight and fat. You can follow a few of his fat loss experiments by going to his website - www.fitscribbler.com - where you will find photos and images of his body transformations.

Andy also writes and creates health and fitness books and at present he has a collection of books which focus on particular areas of womens' wellbeing as well as a number of muscle building books for men. You can find these on his website too.

When he is not working he trains on the beach, cycles, swims, reads, rollerblades and does whatever he can to keep any negative thoughts at bay.

"We have more control over our lives than we think. The sooner we realize this the better the chances are of reaching our goals and fulfilling our dreams" - Andy.

Check out Andy's author website for news on newly released books and special offers:

Fit Scribbler: http://www.fitscribbler.com

Follow Andy on Pinterest: http://www.pinterest.com/fitcribbler

Follow Andy on Twitter at: http://twitter.com/FitScribbler

Follow Andy on Facebook: https://www.facebook.com/fit.scribbler

Follow Andy on Linkedin: http://www.linkedin.com/in/fitscribbler
http://www.linkedin.com/in/fitscribbler

Printed in Great Britain
by Amazon.co.uk, Ltd.,
Marston Gate.